Health Consequences

of Abuse in the Family

Application and Practice in Health Psychology Series

Health Consequences

of Abuse in the Family

A Clinical Guide for Evidence-Based Practice

Edited by
Kathleen A. Kendall-Tackett

American Psychological Association
Washington, DC

Published by
American Psychological Association
750 First Street, NE
Washington, DC 20002
www.apa.org

To order
APA Order Department
P.O. Box 92984
Washington, DC 20090-2984
Tel: (800) 374-2721
Direct: (202) 336-5510
Fax: (202) 336-5502
TDD/TTY: (202) 336-6123
Online: www.apa.org/books/
E-mail: order@apa.org

In the U.K., Europe, Africa, and the Middle East, copies may be ordered from
American Psychological Association
3 Henrietta Street
Covent Garden, London
WC2E 8LU England

Typeset in Goudy by World Composition Services, Inc., Sterling, VA

Printer: Edwards Brothers, Inc., Ann Arbor, MI
Cover Designer: Naylor Design, Washington, DC
Technical/Production Editor: Dan Brachtesende

The opinions and statements published are the responsibility of the authors, and such opinions and statements do not necessarily represent the policies of the American Psychological Association.

Library of Congress Cataloging-in-Publication Data
Health consequences of abuse in the family : a clinical guide for evidence-based practice / edited by Kathleen A. Kendall-Tackett.—1st ed.
p. cm.—(Application and practice in health psychology)
Includes bibliographical references and indexes.
ISBN 1-59147-045-5 (alk. paper)
1. Abused children—Mental health. 2. Adult child abuse victims—Mental health. 3. Family violence—Psychological aspects. 4. Evidence-based psychiatry. I. Kendall-Tackett, Kathleen A. II. Series.

RJ507.A29H43 2004
616.85'822—dc22   2003052339

British Library Cataloguing-in-Publication Data
A CIP record is available from the British Library.

Printed in the United States of America
First Edition

CONTENTS

CONTRIBUTORS

Robert F. Anda, MD, MS, Division of Adult and Community Health, Centers for Disease Control and Prevention, Atlanta, GA

L. Rene Bergeron, MSW, PhD, Department of Social Work, University of New Hampshire, Durham

Amy M. Combs-Lane, PhD, Department of Behavioral Medicine and Psychiatry, West Virginia University School of Medicine, Morgantown

Joanne L. Davis, PhD, Department of Psychology, University of Tulsa, OK

Leonard Diller, PhD, Rusk Institute of Rehabilitation Medicine, New York University Medical Center, New York

Shanta R. Dube, MS, Division of Adult and Community Health, Centers for Disease Control and Prevention, Atlanta, GA

Valerie J. Edwards, PhD, Division of Adult and Community Health, Centers for Disease Control and Prevention, Atlanta, GA

Vincent J. Felitti, MD, Kaiser Permanente, Southern California Permanente Group, San Diego, CA

L. Kevin Hamberger, PhD, Department of Family and Community Medicine, Medical College of Wisconsin, Racine

Sherry L. Hamby, PhD, Possible Equalities, Laurinburg, NC

Debra Pilling Hastings, PhD, RN, CNOR, Dartmouth-Hitchcock Medical Center, Lebanon, NH

Terri J. Haven, MSW, LICSW, private practice, West Springfield, MA

Deborah Issokson, PsyD, Counseling for Reproductive Health and Healing, Watertown, MA

Helene Jackson, PhD, School of Social Work, Columbia University, New York

Glenda Kaufman Kantor, PhD, Family Research Laboratory, University of New Hampshire, Durham

Kathleen A. Kendall-Tackett, PhD, Family Research Laboratory, University of New Hampshire, Durham

Catherine Koverola, PhD, Department of Pediatrics, School of Medicine, University of Maryland, Baltimore

Liza Little, PsyD, RN, Department of Nursing, University of New Hampshire, Durham

Mary W. Meagher, PhD, Department of Psychology, Texas A&M University, College Station

Ronald L. Nuttall, PhD, Lynch School of Education, Boston College, Boston, MA

Subadra Panchanadeswaran, MSW, School of Social Work, University of Maryland, College Park

Darshana Patel, MD, Department of Family and Community Medicine, Medical College of Wisconsin, Racine

Laurie Anne Pearlman, PhD, Traumatic Stress Institute/Center for Adult and Adolescent Psychotherapy, LLC, Trauma Research, Education, and Training Institute, Inc., South Windsor, CT

Elizabeth Philip, MSW, School of Social Work, Columbia University, New York

Jane Rysberg, PhD, Department of Psychology, California State University, Chico

Daniel W. Smith, PhD, National Crime Victims Research and Treatment Center, Medical University of South Carolina, Charleston

SERIES FOREWORD

Division 38 (Health Psychology) of the American Psychological Association presents a new volume in its series focusing on the application and practice of health psychology that examines the relationship between family violence and health issues. One of the primary objectives of the division has been an ongoing interest in health promotion, disease prevention, and treatment through application of principles and procedures that have emerged in the research arena. The vitality of health psychology depends on an active dialogue between researchers and practitioners and the interdependence between the scientific and the applied aspects of the discipline. A primary goal of this series is to continue to expand this dialogue. Accordingly, attempts to translate research findings into applications and interventions, to test and evaluate the effectiveness of these interventions with patient populations, and to denote important clinical experiences and research needs of the practice of health psychology are important foci of these volumes.

It is intended that the volumes in this series will serve as vehicles for translating research into practice, with an analysis of issues related to the evaluation, prevention, and treatment of health behaviors and health problems. These goals are met by conceptualizing clinical and applied health psychology as broadly as possible, including community and public health assessment and intervention methods and problems of health care use. Topics are covered across a wide variety of applied and practice settings, such as hospitals, the practitioner's office, community clinics, the work site, and school environments. Each volume provides direction in areas of need and populations to be served by health psychology intervention. After identifying the population, each volume critically examines issues and problems involved in clinical evaluation, prevention, and treatment of specific disorders and illustrates the effectiveness of clinical approaches to prevention, diagnosis, and treatment that may guide future research and practice. Each volume focuses on seminal topics, such as this book's emphasis on violence and health, and synthesizes research from a range of areas to reinforce the theoretical and scientific rationale for the practice of health psychology.

Dawn K. Wilson and Perry M. Nicassio,
Series Editors

VOLUME FOREWORD

GERALD P. KOOCHER

Too often, health and mental health professionals fall into bifurcated categories with respect to family violence: those with blinders and those with attitude. Chapter 2 provides a superb example of those with blinders: practitioners who ignore, overlook, or simply go about their business oblivious to the reality of domestic abuse in the lives of those for whom they care. Examples of professionals with attitude abound, especially in the popular press, media sound bites, and "advocacy" circles. Such practitioners tend toward zealotry with definite unambiguous knowledge about absolutely necessary long-overdue solutions to the abuse they suspect lies behind every human façade. Not infrequently, the zealots include former victims of abuse who quickly classify others as true believers, unwise folks in need of education, or likely perpetrators. Chapter authors strip away blinders using scientific data, best practices, and thoughtful clinical guidance. Kathleen A. Kendall-Tackett and her interdisciplinary band of experts focus on what we genuinely know from behavioral science and carry us forward to clinical relevance with firm foundation rather than shrill advocacy.

Much of the material across chapters in this volume calls to mind the social psychology literature on bystander intervention. We know that strangers will intervene to help a person in distress when (a) they notice a problem situation, (b) they comprehend the situation as one necessitating an intervention, and (c) they accept a personal responsibility to act. We also know that one reason bystanders may not act relates to uncertainty regarding the best course of action. These factors are well illustrated in the discussions of why health care professionals may not inquire or intervene regarding potential domestic abuse. The guidance offered by Hamberger and

xi

Patel in chapter 4 goes a long way toward overcoming inertia about inquiry and intervention.

Other chapter authors do a superb job of highlighting the needs and vulnerabilities of particular subpopulations, such as ethnic minorities, older people, and individuals with disabilities. In addition, by highlighting the interaction between abuse and certain physical conditions (e.g., traumatic brain injury, pregnancy, and chronic pain), they heighten awareness of the special attention needed in evaluating such patients. The most valuable chapters for practitioners who are able to shed their blinders about domestic and childhood abuse focus on the aftereffects. Recognizing and understanding the sequelae of abuse, as they manifest themselves in health care settings, and crafting strategies to improve the health behavior of current and former victims, constitute the greatest value to this volume.

Readers will want to pay special attention to the chapters addressing the health effects of childhood abuse and neglect. Too often the primary focus in child protection cases zooms in on assessment and protection in the context of specific incidents. What happens later? What are the long-term risks of childhood victimization? How do traumatic events of childhood translate themselves into adult health and quality-of-life issues? Chapters 9 through 13 provide a wealth of guidance on what to expect and how to frame preventive interventions. This compilation provides unique and definitive information for researchers and practitioners alike.

Kathleen A. Kendall-Tackett and her colleagues have accomplished a significant feat by identifying family violence as a genuine public health problem and by presenting an array of strategies to teach about, identify, assess, and intervene with people affected by this major societal issue. They have done so with sensitivity, scholarship, wise clinical guidance, and scientific rigor in a manner unique for writings on such topics. Their work will inspire informed advocacy driven by data, rather than polemics, and education based on evidence rather than affect.

ACKNOWLEDGMENTS

This book exists because of the efforts of a large number of people. First, I would like to thank the chapter authors who contributed to this book. I had high expectations for your work, and you exceeded them. Thank you for all you do on behalf of children and families.

Margaret Chesney deserves a special thanks. Margaret served as midwife for this project, guiding it from idea, to book proposal, to final project. I could not have done it without you.

Dawn Wilson served as encourager at that crucial midpoint, where enthusiasm was lagging. It really helped. Jerry Suls and Andy Baum have also been supportive and helpful at several steps along the way. Thanks so much for your feedback, comments, and suggestions.

Susan Reynolds at the American Psychological Association has been a pleasure to work with. She has answered my many questions and shared from the wisdom of her experience. Kristine Enderle also provided lots of helpful feedback at the critical midpoint edit. This feedback helped us pull together the chapters to create a whole.

Paula Schnurr shares my passion for understanding the health impact of traumatic events. She generously shared the outline of the book she and Bonnie Green were editing so that, among the three of us, we covered the topic thoroughly but did not overlap. Thanks for your collegial spirit.

I would also like to thank my colleagues David Finkelhor and Murray Straus at the Family Research Laboratory and Crimes Against Children Research Center for inspiring excellence in all that you do. Also, I extend many thanks to the staff of the Family Violence Research Conferences— Sarah Giacomoni, Doreen Cole, Kelly Foster, and Vicki Benn—for holding down the fort while I was off working on another book.

Finally, to my own family I say thank you for allowing me the space and time I needed to edit this book. I appreciate your love and support, even as you had to endure months of mom with "book brain."

Health Consequences

of Abuse in the Family

INTRODUCTION: FAMILY VIOLENCE AS A HEALTH ISSUE

KATHLEEN A. KENDALL-TACKETT

Each year, millions of men, women, and children are beaten, raped, or assaulted by members of their own families (American Medical Association, 1995; Tjaden & Thoennes, 2000). The statistics are so overwhelming that three major health organizations—the Centers for Disease Control (2001), the American Medical Association (1995), and the World Health Organization (1999, 2002)—have identified family violence as a major threat to public health.

INTERSECTION OF FAMILY VIOLENCE AND HEALTH

The majority of reports on family violence and health have focused on immediate consequences, such as injury. And these needs are substantial. According to the National Violence Against Women Survey, 39% of female victims of violence reported injuries. In a single year, approximately 500,000 women sought medical care for their injuries, and 62% of these women were seen in emergency departments (Tjaden & Thoennes, 2000). Family-violence-related injury leads to massive demands on the health care system.

However, researchers are increasingly beginning to understand that injuries represent the tip of the iceberg in terms of health effects. Indeed, the health care needs of people who have experienced previous family violence may vastly overwhelm the numbers of people who are seeking assistance for current injuries. Family violence has been related to a wide range of chronic diseases and conditions, including chronic pain, ischemic heart disease, cancer, stroke, chronic bronchitis, emphysema, diabetes, skeletal fractures, and hepatitis (Felitti et al., 2001; Kendall-Tackett & Marshall, 1999).

It is not surprising that survivors of family violence have high rates of health care use. They make more visits to primary care physicians, specialists, and emergency departments. They report more symptoms, have more procedures and diagnostic tests, and have surgery more often. Yet they are often very unhappy with the care they receive, and they may indeed be retraumatized by their health care providers (Kendall-Tackett, 2003).

ROLE OF MENTAL HEALTH PROVIDERS

Psychologists and other mental health providers have been at the forefront of treatment for victims and survivors of family violence. Despite this, a curious schism exists. Psychologists are often well equipped to treat depression or posttraumatic stress disorder but have left their clients' physical health to medical providers. Indeed, mental health professionals often overlook, or even allegorize, physical health complaints.

ABOUT THIS BOOK

The chapters in this book represent the cutting edge in a new area of study within the family violence field. In this book, the chapter authors have used a scientist–practitioner model. Each chapter summarizes the latest research and offers practical suggestions for what mental health professionals can do. Although mental health providers are the primary audience, the chapter authors themselves represent a wide range of health professions, including medicine, nursing, and social work. I anticipate that this book will be helpful to a wide variety of health care professionals.

Throughout this volume, the chapter authors present case descriptions of reports. Some of these cases are composites of situations and patients the authors have encountered in their clinical work. Other cases are descriptions of particular patients, with all names and other identifying information changed to protect their identities and preserve confidentiality.

The first chapter provides an overview of family violence and describes some of the unique issues involved in working with this population in a health care setting. After that, the chapters are grouped into two main parts. The chapters in the first part deal with screening for various types of family violence in health care settings. The chapters in the second part deal with some of the more common symptoms of past and current abuse, including chronic pain, high-risk behavior, dissociation, childbearing difficulties, and traumatic brain injury. For some topics, and some populations, the coverage may seem incomplete. That reflects the state of the field. As with any emerging field, the knowledge base is not yet complete. Even in this instance, however, the chapter authors were able to fill in the gaps with their considerable clinical experience.

CONCLUSION

The health effects of family violence offer mental and medical health care providers an opportunity to work together. Without a collaborative approach, many of these patients will fall through the cracks. They might respond by becoming "difficult" or by simply refusing to seek medical treatment. Using a team approach, psychologists can identify families caught in the web of violence, guide patients to appropriate resources, and save both patients and the health care system the cost of unnecessary and unhelpful procedures. It is up to you to decide how you will respond to this rare window of opportunity. The time to act is now.

REFERENCES

American Medical Association. (1995). *Diagnostic and treatment guidelines on the mental health effects of family violence*. Retrieved November 15, 2001, from http://www.ama-assn.org

Centers for Disease Control. (2001). *Intimate partner violence fact sheet*. Retrieved June 10, 2002, from http://www.cdc.org/nationalcenterforinjuryprevention

Felitti, V. J., Anda, R. F., Nordenberg, D., Williamson, D. F., Spitz, A. M., Edwards, V., et al. (2001). Relationship of childhood abuse and household dysfunction to many of the leading causes of death in adults. In K. Franey, R. Geffner, & R. Falconer (Eds.), *The cost of child maltreatment: Who pays? We all do* (pp. 53–69). San Diego, CA: Family Violence and Sexual Assault Institute.

Kendall-Tackett, K. A. (2003). *Treating the long-term health effects of childhood abuse: A guide for mental health, medical and social service professionals*. New York: Civic Research Institute.

Kendall-Tackett, K. A., & Marshall, R. (1999). Victimization and diabetes: An exploratory study. *Child Abuse and Neglect, 23*, 593–596.

Tjaden, P., & Thoennes, N. (2000). *Extent, nature, and consequences of intimate partner violence: Findings from the National Violence Against Women Survey.* Washington, DC: National Institute of Justice.

World Health Organization. (1999, April 8). *WHO recognizes child abuse as a public health problem.* Retrieved June 10, 2002, from http://www.who.org/PR-99-20

World Health Organization. (2002). *Child abuse and neglect.* Retrieved June 10, 2002, from http://www.who.org/violenceandintentionalinjury

1

THE SPECTRUM OF VICTIMIZATION AND THE IMPLICATIONS FOR HEALTH

SHERRY L. HAMBY

People who have suffered one type of abuse are at increased risk of other types. Health care providers need to be familiar with all the various types of family violence and how these can differentially affect health. There are similarities in the dynamics and consequences of different forms of family violence that are also useful to recognize. I offer practical suggestions for intervention and describe legal obligations of psychologists and other health care professionals, use of diagnostic categories to record information in medical records, and protection of patient confidentiality.

A patient has been referred to your mental health clinic in a large public hospital because she has asked for help in stopping smoking. She had previously unsuccessfully tried a nicotine patch product and has now been given a prescription for Zyban, also known as the antidepressant Wellbutrin (buproprion). You start her on a cognitive–behavioral smoking cessation program. She attends only a handful of therapy sessions. A few weeks later, her physician approaches you because this patient has asked for a renewal of her Zyban prescription but also reported that she has not stopped smoking and has given up on the smoking cessation program. He wonders why she wants the antidepressant if she is not attempting to quit smoking. He also reports that this woman has no significant health problems but nonetheless presents to his office fairly regularly with a variety of minor concerns.

How well you can answer the physician's question depends in part on your familiarity with the spectrum of family violence and how victimization-related symptoms can manifest in health care settings. A woman might seek antidepressants for numerous reasons, but ongoing or past abuse is one of the most likely. Did you screen for the presence of abuse in your initial assessment? Did you ask about all the major forms of abuse, or just one? Did you ascertain whether the patient is experiencing any symptoms that could be the sequelae of trauma? Is she concerned about the safety of her children, parents, or other family members? Did you recognize high medical utilization as a common consequence of family violence?

In today's health care world there are contradictory pressures to provide high-quality care and to provide it to increasingly greater numbers of patients. Family violence is one of the most common problems confronted by adults and children alike; it is more common than psychotic symptoms, suicidal ideation, or a variety of other issues for which mental health professionals more routinely screen in psychological assessments. A basic level of knowledge about the spectrum of family violence is an important and efficient tool for providing better quality care. Instead of becoming a treatment dropout, the patient described above could become a treatment success with an appropriate intervention that takes into account the full context of her family situation.

THE SPECTRUM OF FAMILY VICTIMIZATION

Family violence is an umbrella term that refers to many forms of abuse, including partner violence (also called *domestic violence*), child abuse and neglect, elder abuse, and sexual assault. Each of these specific forms is associated with numerous health and mental health consequences; what is less appreciated is that there are many similarities in the consequences and the hypothesized mechanisms for those consequences across forms of family violence. Furthermore, there is increasing evidence of a significant amount of overlap among these forms. Most estimates of the overlap of partner violence and child abuse in the same home are in the 30% to 60% range (Edleson, 1999). In one large study, neglect specifically was found to have a 24% overlap with partner violence (Trocme et al., 2001). Approximately 26% to 52% of women who have been beaten by male partners have also been raped (Koss, Ingram, & Pepper, 1997). Revictimization of the same individual also is common. Women who were abused as children are at elevated risk for experiencing partner violence and sexual assault as adults (Kaufman Kantor & Jasinski, 1998; Koss & Dinero, 1989). Some elder abuse is partner violence that has persisted into the victim's later years (National Center on Elder Abuse, 1998).

Family violence also includes other forms of violence, such as sibling assault and abuse of family members who are vulnerable because of physical or cognitive incapacity. Information is unfortunately limited on sibling assault, child assault of nonelderly parents, assaults of adult family members with disabilities, and other forms (Hamby & Finkelhor, 2000). It is also worth noting that the term *family* is construed broadly in family violence research. For example, *partner violence* usually refers not only to spouses but also to girlfriends, boyfriends, or other intimate partners, including same-sex partners. Perpetrators of child abuse can be anyone in a caregiving role, including stepparents, live-in nonmarital partners, grandparents, or others.

All of the major forms of family violence have significant implications for health care provision. Health care settings as diverse as emergency departments, primary-care practices, gastroenterology departments, pediatric clinics, radiology departments, surgery centers, and obstetrical care clinics all see high numbers of family violence victims (Hamby & Koss, 2003). Basic information for providers is offered in this chapter and summarized in Exhibit 1.1. A broad perspective that identifies similarities while also acknowledging differences can be an efficient method of organizing knowledge on dynamics and interventions.

CONSEQUENCES OF FAMILY VIOLENCE SEEN IN HEALTH CARE SETTINGS

Many of the chapters in this book examine in detail the health consequences for various victim groups. Here, I present an overview that emphasizes similarities and differences in health care consequences across all of the forms of family violence.

Health Consequences Common to All Forms of Family Violence

One of the most important health consequences seen among all victims of family violence is increased medical utilization. *Increased medical utilization* refers to the average number of physician visits over a year or some other fixed period of time. Research has shown not only that abuse victims see physicians more frequently but also that this increase does *not* occur prior to the violence, and it holds even after eliminating visits due to assault injuries (Kimerling & Calhoun, 1994).

EXHIBIT 1.1
What Health Care Providers Should Know About the Spectrum of Victimization

✓ The spectrum of family victimization includes partner violence, child abuse and neglect, elder abuse, and sexual assault. It also includes less recognized forms such as sibling assault and assault of family members with disabilities.

✓ There is a significant degree of overlap among child abuse, partner violence, and sexual assault in the same home, with most estimates ranging from 24% to 60%. Multiple forms of abuse should not be assumed, however.

✓ Health care settings as diverse as emergency departments, primary-care practices, gastroenterology departments, pediatric clinics, radiology departments, surgery centers, and obstetrical care clinics all see high numbers of family violence victims.

✓ Mandatory reporting obligations for child abuse, elder abuse, and partner violence should be disclosed early in any clinical interview. Providers should be familiar with their own state laws and know which categories of victim require mandatory reporting.

✓ Vulnerable family members need privacy and protection from the perpetrator during the initial screening and subsequent interviews. Adult patients should be allowed to designate what medical information will be disclosed and to whom it will be disclosed.

✓ Assessments should inquire about all major forms of family violence, not just one or two. Systematic screenings yield much more disclosures than informal reports.

✓ There may be more than one victim in a household.

✓ There may be victims who are unknown to your patient.

✓ Participation on a coordinated community response team is the best-established method of interagency communication and has been shown to improve services to victims.

✓ Documentation of contacts with victims of violence are often subpoenaed for criminal cases and for civil cases, including those pertaining to custody of children, divorce, and competency or power of attorney. Records can also be needed to qualify for exemptions to welfare rules.

✓ Mental health documentation should follow the patient's report closely, emphasize behavioral descriptions, and avoid victim blaming.

✓ Many patients, especially adult victims of childhood abuse, may wish to protect their privacy as much as provide documentation of the victimization. It is important to be sensitive to patients' wishes for privacy and not to provide access to mental health notes to more providers than is absolutely necessary.

✓ Family violence has many dynamics that are common across forms of violence. These include perpetrator power that arises out of the family role the perpetrator holds, easy access to family victims, and betrayal of family trust.

✓ Children and adults with cognitive impairment may lack the legal standing or cognitive skills needed to assist in protecting themselves from violence.

✓ Parents of minor age children may be more vulnerable to violence because they fear losing custody of their children.

✓ Witnessing/indirect victimization is another way that trauma affects entire families. Two of the most important forms are witnessing domestic violence and secondary trauma that affects family members of people who have suffered through war or oppression.

(continued)

EXHIBIT 1.1   *(Continued)*

✓ Increased medical utilization, traumatic injury, death, chronic pain, and gastrointestinal disorders have been documented in survivors of many forms of family violence.

✓ Sexual assault victims may experience unique sequelae, including pregnancy, sexually transmitted diseases, subsequent fear of sex, arousal dysfunction, and decreased sexual interest.

✓ Abused pregnant women are at risk for a variety of adverse effects on fetuses and may have limited access to prenatal care.

✓ Neglected and abused children may experience impaired brain development through the effects of stress or malnutrition. Neglected children are at risk for academic underachievement that may have lasting consequences.

✓ Family violence is one of the most common problems confronted by adults and children alike; it is more common than psychotic symptoms, suicidal ideation, or a variety of other issues for which mental health professionals more routinely screen in psychological assessments. A basic knowledge about the spectrum of family violence is an important and efficient tool to providing better quality health care.

Of course, traumatic injury is higher among victims of family violence than among members of the general population. This also includes death. There are many less obvious consequences of family victimization, however. Various types of chronic pain, including chronic pelvic pain, headache, and irritable bowel syndrome, are more common among victimized than nonvictimized women.

Health Consequences Unique to Specific Forms of Family Violence

Although there are many consequences that are similar across forms of violence, there are also important, unique outcomes. Violence that involves sexual activity includes the risks of sexual activity as well as the risks of physical harm. Some groups are vulnerable for specific consequences because of their developmental stage. These include women of childbearing age and children.

Sexual Assault and Rape

Sexual assault has perhaps the greatest number of specific health consequences. Pregnancy itself is a direct consequence of about 5% of all rapes (Holmes, Resnick, Kilpatrick, & Best, 1996). Almost half (47%) of rapes leading to pregnancy were perpetrated by a husband or boyfriend. Women who experience forced sex are also at high risk for contracting sexually transmitted diseases of all types (Goodman, Koss, & Russo, 1993). This includes women who are forced into having sex without a condom, a common but often overlooked type of sexual coercion. In addition, victims of sexual assault, including a childhood history of sexual trauma, are at risk for experiencing subsequent fear of sex, arousal dysfunction, and decreased sexual interest (Goodman et al., 1993; Mahoney & Williams, 1998).

Assault of Women of Childbearing Age

Women in the childbearing years are at risk for adverse effects of violence on pregnancy and in some cases even the ability to bear children. Several studies have shown that violence likely has an adverse effect on the fetus, although there are so many factors that contribute to pregnancy outcome research that the findings have been mixed. Some adverse effects that have been found are that abused women are more likely than nonabused women to show low maternal weight gain, have more infections, experience preterm labor, and deliver low-birthweight infants (Berenson, Wiemann, Wilkinson, Jones, & Anderson, 1994; Parker, McFarlane, & Soeken, 1994; Schei, Samuelson, & Bakketeig, 1991; Shumway et al., 1999). Some studies have found that women who have experienced abuse are more likely to delay receiving prenatal care until the third trimester, possibly because of interference from the batterer (McFarlane, Parker, Soeken, & Bullock, 1992; Parker et al., 1994). In a study of pregnant trauma patients, 29% of trauma-related perinatal deaths were due to domestic violence (Connolly, Katz, Bash, McMahon, & Hansen, 1997). Violence appears to be a significantly more common problem among pregnant women than a variety of other conditions that are already included in most routine screenings during pregnancy, such as pre-eclampsia, gestational diabetes, and placenta previa (Gazmararian et al., 1996).

Child Abuse and Neglect

Normal childhood development of brain and body functions can be impaired because of abuse. Recent research is beginning to outline actual neurobiological effects of abuse that are distinct from traumatic injury. For example, a recent study suggests that individuals with a childhood abuse history may have impaired development of the cerebellar vermis, a limbic system structure that affects an individual's ability to regulate irritability in the limbic system. Limbic system irritability may be a risk factor for substance abuse and other problems (Anderson, Teicher, Polcari, & Renshaw, 2002).

Neglect has numerous health consequences that are generally underappreciated by providers. Children who are medically neglected and do not receive their vaccinations are at greater risk for a variety of serious childhood diseases, such as measles. Neglected children often suffer from malnutrition and its associated consequences. Unlike victims of other forms of family violence, they may suffer more from medical underutilization than overutilization. Neglected children often are absent from school more than other youth and as a result may have long-term problems with cognitive and academic achievement (Kendall-Tackett & Eckenrode, 1997).

ASSESSMENT: IDENTIFYING VICTIMS IN NEED

Ethical and Safety Issues to Address in the First Interview

Privacy and confidentiality are two of the most important ethical issues for family violence intervention. Many privacy and confidentiality considerations are the same as for any therapy patient. These include providing a private environment; clearly communicating confidentiality guidelines; and specifying whether parents of juveniles, other providers, or insurance companies will have access to any treatment information. There are several ethical issues that are unique to family violence.

Disclose Mandatory Reporting Obligations

Disclose as early as possible your mandatory reporting obligations to child protective services, adult protective services, and the police. This includes explaining not only state mandatory reporting laws but also the policies of your hospital or clinic. Some emergency departments routinely report to the police incidents that appear to be crimes. It is critically important that patients do not feel betrayed when mandatory reporting requirements dictate that you break confidentiality. Patients who feel further victimized by mental health providers can easily fall off the radar of all community services unless a serious abuse-related medical emergency arises. Providers should not count on social services agencies to order treatment when the willingness to participate in treatment voluntarily is lost. It is estimated that only 40% to 60% of child protective services cases receive services after the investigation (Edleson, in press).

Privacy and Protection From the Perpetrator

It may seem surprising, but victims of family violence are still frequently interviewed in semiprivate or public environments—or, worse, in the presence of the probable perpetrator. Not long ago, I was called to an emergency clinic to talk with a woman who had been stabbed in the abdomen by her husband. Her wounds were sufficiently serious that she was transferred from our rural clinic to a major urban medical center. The medical staff who interviewed my patient asked her husband to leave the hospital room, but they did not close the door. He stood slightly outside the door, glared at the victim and shook his head "no" every time they asked her who had hurt her or whether she wanted any restrictions on visitation. His threats were successful, and she did not identify him as the perpetrator or request visitation limits. As a consequence, the social worker did not implement the hospital's abuse protocol (despite the documentation that arrived with the woman from our clinic) and allowed her husband free access to her and her medical information during her stay, including her discharge date and time. He picked her up from the hospital and took her home, where she was eventually able to contact me. At that point, I had lost credibility along with the hospital staff because I had assured her they would help her when she arrived at the hospital. She returned to the clinic not to ask for further assistance but to express anger at the failure of the system. She declined further intervention.

A private room with no traffic from other patients or providers is the best environment for an interview. At a minimum, all trauma victims should be interviewed alone, away from family members, no matter how helpful or concerned intimate partners, parents, or other family members may appear. In emergency departments that still use curtains to separate beds (an arrangement that is still in place in the hospital that serves the rural county where I live), moving to another area of the hospital may be necessary. Victims who require inpatient treatment should be able to provide a list of people who may receive information about their care over the phone or in person. Mechanisms should be in place to facilitate the use of this list by personnel working all three hospital shifts. The discharge plan, in particular, can be a highly sensitive piece of information in cases of family violence. Victims who wish to be discharged to a domestic violence shelter or older adult community residence may be unable to do so if the perpetrator shows up at the designated discharge time.

Comprehensive Assessments Ask About All Major Forms of Victimization

A good treatment plan requires a thorough assessment of violence experiences. Screening for violence has increased in many hospitals but is still far from universal. Many private clinics still assess violence histories sporadically, if at all. There are comprehensive assessment tools for youth (Hamby & Finkelhor, 2001). For adults, fewer broad-spectrum tools are available, but there are a number that measure male partner violence and sexual assault (e.g., Straus, Hamby, Boney-McCoy, & Sugarman, 1996; Tjaden & Thoennes, 2000). Detailed questioning leads to fuller disclosure of abuse (Bolen & Scannapieco, 1999). Nonetheless, even minimal systematic screening in health care settings greatly improves identification over informal recordkeeping (McLeer & Anwar, 1989).

Virtually all clinicians are aware that there are many situations in which such an assessment has the potential to greatly complicate their work. If a patient is an adult woman who is a victim of partner violence, in most states (but not all) a mental health professional would be under no obligation to report those incidents to protective services or law enforcement. That is not the case for children or elderly victims, however. Thus it is extremely important that mental health professionals understand their state's reporting obligations. The definitions of *abuse* and *maltreatment* vary from state to state, and the type of victims (children, elderly, and partners) who must be reported varies also. The nature, extent, and quality of protective services and law enforcement intervention vary tremendously also (Edleson, in press; Hamby & Finkelhor, 2000). It is important to be familiar with the agencies and their staff in one's area and to work with protective services agencies to provide maximum safety and benefit to victims. Participation in a coordinated community response team (described later in this chap.) is one excellent means of coordinating services for the maximum benefit of victims.

There Can Be Many Victims in One Household

In dealing with victims, it is important to recognize that the victim in front of you may not be the only one. Witnessing domestic violence is a separate issue from assaults that specifically target children, but this should also be considered. It is not known what the rate of overlap is between elder abuse and other forms of family violence, but if there is an elderly person in the home, then that possibility should be considered as well. The frequency of overlap indicates that a thorough assessment of a family situation involves ascertaining the family composition and asking about the victimization experiences of all family members. As stated earlier, such an assessment should be conducted after mandatory reporting obligations have been disclosed.

Perpetrators May Commit Offenses Against Victims Who Are Unknown to Each Other

Perpetrators may have victims outside the family of the victim who is known to you. In cases of partner violence, many times there are multiple relationships in which the batterer has acted violently. This information is important for risk assessments and safety planning because it suggests a greater likelihood of ongoing violence (e.g., Kropp, Hart, Webster, & Eaves, 1995). For providers working with adult victims, risk assessment may be the only reason for determining whether there are other adult victims. With juvenile victims, however, the possibility of other victims does raise mandatory reporting issues, even when the current child is not perceived to be in danger. This is especially true in cases of family perpetrators of sexual abuse who are noncaregivers.

Many times I have heard from colleagues or patients about incidents in which a child was assaulted by a relative outside the immediate family, typically an older cousin or uncle. Parents naturally tend to focus on their own children's safety and usually protect their child from further assault by keeping the child away from the perpetrator. Often they do not report the assault at the time, and it is frequently as much as a year or two later before the incident is disclosed, often because the child shows signs of posttraumatic stress. Parents are often worried, frequently with good cause, about the stigma of becoming a publicly known victim of sexual assault, and may be reluctant to report sexual offenses, especially in cases where they feel able to prevent further incidents. Parents are also often understandably concerned about the response of relatives, such as the spouse or parent of the alleged perpetrator.

Many providers are sympathetic to these concerns and wonder whether reporting is mandated if the child appears to be in no imminent danger. Child protective cases are often complicated and messy, and some providers are reluctant to report unless it seems absolutely necessary. There are unfortunately still many jurisdictions in which the law enforcement response to such incidents creates further distress for the victim. Nonetheless, it is important to consider that, from a public health standpoint, the issue of protection extends not only to the known victim but also to other potential victims. Few state mandatory reporting laws permit a psychologist to make a personal judgment about the appropriate intervention in these cases. Moreover, few state laws make reference to judgments about imminent danger, and most require reporting whenever there is reasonable suspicion that abuse has occurred. The offender may well have assaulted other victims. If the offender is also a juvenile, he may also be a victim in need of protection. In either case, the offender is probably in need of interventions that will protect other children and also provide therapeutic help for him.

WORKING WITH COORDINATED COMMUNITY RESPONSE TEAMS

Violence is a social ill as well as a psychological issue. Unlike some psychological issues, violence needs to be addressed at both the community and the individual level. In many communities, there are several mechanisms in place to do this. One of the most effective of these is called the *coordinated community response* (CCR) *model*, which is associated with its place of origin in Duluth, Minnesota (Shepard & Pence, 1999). The CCR model involves interagency communication among health care providers, domestic violence advocates, child protective service workers, police officers, court personnel, and others who often respond to family violence. It is no secret that these various social agencies typically have different institutional missions and cultures and, many times, widely varying attitudes toward victims of violence (Pence, 1999). It is not unusual for these agencies to have distant if not hostile relationships in a community. Victims often suffer as a result, as they get treated differently by different professionals, sometimes advised in contradictory directions, and receive little assistance in negotiating the various bureaucracies. However, an active effort to coordinate interagency responses that focuses on interdisciplinary discussion of specific cases can make real improvements in this system (Hamby, 1998; Shepard & Pence, 1999).

The CCR model is primarily identified with domestic violence but could be expanded to include other forms of family violence. Hospitals with emergency departments are probably the most important health care institutions that should be involved in a CCR. It is not necessary for all psychologists affiliated with a hospital or clinic to participate on a CCR team, but someone who is familiar with the institution's policies and staff, and who sees patients experiencing family violence, should be a regular member. Obstetrical clinics or other health care facilities that see high numbers of family violence victims could also benefit from participation on a CCR team. In most communities, domestic violence shelters or community centers are key organizers of CCR teams, and contacting them should provide information about how to participate.

DOCUMENTATION ISSUES IN HEALTH AND MENTAL HEALTH CARE

Diagnostic labels and the content of medical records are often of great concern to past and current victims of family violence, who are often confronted with conflicting needs. On the one hand, many victims will want to thoroughly document incidents, not only to receive adequate health care but also to provide legal documentation. On the other hand, many victims experience considerable shame and stigma and want to protect their privacy as much as possible. They view written medical records as one of the greatest threats to that privacy.

Legal Uses of Mental Health and Medical Documentation

Patients with victimization histories are probably among the most likely to have their records subpoenaed for legal proceedings. These proceedings can include not only criminal prosecution of the perpetrator but also custody, divorce, and competency or power-of-attorney hearings. Documentation is also important for victims applying for welfare assistance, as battered women are entitled to certain exemptions from welfare requirements (Raphael, 1999).

It can be extremely helpful to victims to identify these possible needs. Mental health records should follow patients' reports closely, focus on behavioral descriptions, and avoid drawing unnecessary conclusions about circumstances of incidents. Defense attorneys sometimes adopt a strategy of blaming the victim to reduce the culpability of their patient, and the contents of mental health records should not include information that could be interpreted as victim blaming. If a patient has been previously seen, any increase or change in posttraumatic stress or other symptoms after an assault is important to note. If the evidence supports it, it is helpful to make connections between the patient's symptoms and her or his trauma history. For example, posttraumatic stress disorder and acute stress disorder explicate this relationship more effectively than borderline personality disorder or many of the anxiety or depressive disorders (American Psychiatric Association, 1994). The V Codes for Problems Related to Abuse and Neglect (American Psychiatric Association, 1994) are often appropriate diagnoses, especially in situations where a psychologist is consulting to a medical team that is treating physical injuries and signs of psychological distress do not meet criteria for an Axis I disorder. The V codes also have the advantage of being less stigmatizing than Axis I disorders. There have been anecdotal reports of perpetrator's attempting to use a victim's distress after abuse as evidence of her unfitness to keep custody of her children. Thus, it is important not to overdiagnose a victim's symptoms.

Documentation and Privacy Needs

Notwithstanding the possible need to obtain independent documentation of violence, victims may wish that documentation of their history be minimal in their medical records. Anecdotally, this seems to be especially true of adult survivors of child abuse who are no longer in contact with the perpetrator. (Indeed, in some cases the perpetrator is deceased and there will definitely be no legal action.) People often do not realize that every comment they make to a health care provider can potentially go into their health record. Many patients do not enjoy the option of seeing the same medical provider each time they see a general practitioner, psychiatrist, or other physician. Although it is less likely that a patient's psychologist will change from visit to visit, it is not unusual for a psychologist's records to be available to other members of a treatment team in a health maintenance organization, outpatient clinic, or hospital. On more than one occasion I have had a patient complain that she disclosed an abuse history to one provider whom she trusted, not realizing that the provider would document the abuse in her record. Then, on a subsequent visit, a different provider glanced at her chart and casually commented, "Oh, I see you have an abuse history," much to the dismay of the patient.

Discuss with an adult patient how to document an abuse history. Suggest different options. Some computerized systems allow providers to control how much information will be displayed to other providers when they open a patient's record. If so, consider limiting that information or labeling certain information as confidential or to be discussed only with the approval of the patient. The amount of detail can be limited while still conveying the essential information. Psychologists are also in an excellent position to act as ombudsmen for patients in these situations. Often other medical providers are not aware of the distress they caused and are happy to accommodate the patient's wishes. Some patients may feel more comfortable approaching a psychologist rather than a physician about these issues.

UNIQUE CLINICAL ISSUES FOR DIFFERENT VICTIM GROUPS

Legal issues pertaining to documentation affect many victims. As with the other topics addressed here, however, there are certain classes of victims that have unique legal concerns. Dependents, including not only children but some elderly and cognitively impaired individuals, and guardians of dependents, are two groups that may be limited in their responses to family violence.

Lack of Independent Legal Standing for Children and for Some Elderly and Cognitively Impaired Individuals

Children lack the legal standing and the life skills to care for themselves. They lack authority in almost all of their social roles and are unlikely to be able to increase their own safety. They are largely dependent on other adults, either inside or outside the family, to access interventions for themselves or the perpetrator, or to find an alternate home if necessary.

Some older people, especially those experiencing moderate to severe dementia, have lost legal decision-making power through court proceedings or perhaps voluntary assignment of power of attorney to another person. Most often, legal responsibility is given to another family member. It is obvious that if the family is experiencing violence this can further disadvantage an elderly individual. Individuals who retain mental capacity may still be unable to handle the physical or financial requirements needed to change their living situation or perform their own self-care. There is no system in place that is comparable to the foster care system for children, and without considerable financial resources elderly and disabled individuals may have few options other than institutionalization. Many individuals would prefer to tolerate the abuse than give up home life for institutions, which often would also mean giving up access to friends, familiar neighborhoods, and support systems such as those provided by local churches.

Custody and Other Legal Issues for Parents of Juveniles

Most victims of domestic violence are legally competent but are still constrained by legal issues. For example, they often risk losing custody of their children in divorce proceedings. Instances still occur in which batterers try to charge their wives with kidnapping for taking their children to a shelter. Although these charges are no longer a threat in most criminal courts, they can influence judges in civil divorce proceedings. Mothers of minors are at risk for being charged by child protective agencies for failing to protect their children if their children witness the abuse of their mother. They may be forced to follow the treatment plans of child protective service workers who know little about domestic violence situations.

DYNAMICS OF FAMILY VIOLENCE

To fully understand the spectrum of family violence requires a focus on perpetrators as well as on victims. Many perpetrators are consistently violent over time in many of their intimate relationships. It is important to try to establish this history. Evidence of multiple victims strongly suggests that the violence is part of an ongoing interpersonal strategy, often a sign of serious character disorder rather than a fleeting response to unusually stressful circumstances, as abusers often claim. Perpetrators who have offended against multiple victims have much poorer treatment prognoses and are at greater risk for perpetrating severe violence in the future (Hamby, 1998; Kropp et al., 1995).

Providers in health care settings are more likely to have contact with victims seeking help for injuries or other traumatic sequelae than with perpetrators, who seldom seek treatment voluntarily. A focus on the perpetrator's behavior is, if anything, even more important when working with victims and often is more difficult, as the perpetrator is not the patient. Focusing on the perpetrator's behavior is a way to avoid victim blaming and mistakenly looking for the solution to the violence in victim behavior. It is also essential for helping the victim make a safety plan that corresponds, as much as possible, to the best possible assessment of risk (with a recognition that no risk assessment can be perfectly accurate). The following discussion of dynamics, while focusing on the victim's perspective, nonetheless is primarily informed by an analysis of perpetration.

Commonalties Across the Spectrum of Victimization

Clinicians and researchers focusing on specific forms of family violence have long ago identified numerous ways in which various forms of family assaults are distinct from crimes committed by stranger assailants (e.g., Browne & Finkelhor, 1986; Stanko, 1988). It has only recently been recognized that all forms of family violence, in fact, share many of these features. Three of the most important dynamics pertain to power, access, and betrayal.

Power

Most perpetrators of assault, whether strangers or intimates, are taking advantage of perceived weakness in the victim. In the case of stranger assaults, these weaknesses typically involve either physical disparities between the strength and size of the victim relative to the perpetrator or temporary social isolation (e.g., walking alone at night). Family perpetrators exploit weaknesses, too. Parents are bigger and stronger than children are, at least until children's teen years. Adult children may suddenly find themselves stronger than their elderly parents. Most victims of elder abuse (defined as abuse of anyone over age 60) are age 80 or over, suggesting that growing physical weakness leads to increased vulnerability (National Center on Elder Abuse, 1998). Men are, on average, more than 30 pounds (13.6 kg) heavier, 5 inches (12.7 cm) taller, (National Center for Health Statistics, 1994), and possess 50% more upper body and 30% more lower body strength than the average woman (Powers & Howley, 1997). This physical advantage is one reason why partner assaults of women are more likely to lead to injury than partner assaults of men (Stets & Straus, 1990; Tjaden & Thoennes, 2000).

Family perpetrators have other sources of power, though, that stranger perpetrators do not have. Most family perpetrators have role authority. Parents have the legal authority in every state to physically chastise their children. Senior family members may have once enjoyed the perquisites of family authority but are now vulnerable because of their physical health or the loss of status due to retirement. Men still enjoy significant role authority in marriage and other romantic relationships. They make more money than women (U.S. Bureau of the Census, 2001) and are more likely to be accommodated regarding family schedules and decisions (Fox & Murry, 2000). When violence occurs, or is even threatened, family members who lack power may hesitate to confront the perpetrator lest they find themselves in an even worse situation.

Access

Perpetrators of family violence typically have daily or at least very frequent contact with their victims. In many cases, children, elderly family members, and even spouses are unable to leave the home or otherwise avoid the perpetrator. As a result, family violence often involves chronic trauma that is repeated many times. The repeated nature of family violence is one of its most traumagenic aspects (e.g., Banyard & Hamby, 1996).

Betrayal

Betrayal has been emphasized primarily in the child abuse literature (Browne & Finkelhor, 1986), but it is an important dynamic in all forms of family violence. The family is supposed to be a source of love, nurturance, and support. Family perpetrators violate basic civil guidelines not to harm other citizens and personal bonds of trust. Furthermore, perpetration by family members can be complex and confusing, because it often happens in tandem with more loving acts toward the victim.

Witnessing and Indirect Victimizations

Providers are increasingly broadening their perspective even further and considering the effects of victimization on others in the family. Witnesses and indirect victims do not suffer an actual physical, psychological, or sexual assault themselves but are either present when one occurs or are exposed to the aftermath of such assaults. Witnessing family violence can include incidents such as being present at the murder of a relative and viewing or hearing parental abuse of another child in the family (Hamby & Finkelhor, 1999). Witnessing domestic violence has received the most attention. *Indirect victimization* can refer to any situation when a family member experiences vicarious trauma because of the aftermath of an assault on a family member. Sometimes these effects are immediate, as when a child becomes distressed from seeing his or her mother bruised or injured from partner violence, even though the child was not present during the assault. An important form of indirect victimization is *secondary trauma*, in which the consequences of traumatic events are passed on to children, spouses, and even grandchildren who are far removed in time and place from the initial traumatic event.

Witnessing Domestic Violence

Clinical interest in witnessing domestic violence has mushroomed in recent years. Exposure to domestic violence is associated with depression; anxiety; failure to thrive; sleeplessness; and psychosomatic symptoms, such as bedwetting. The mechanism for these effects can be both direct, from the personal witnessing of abuse, and indirect, from the effects of having a victimized parent who may be physically injured, depressed, or otherwise limited in his or her ability to provide care (Edleson, in press; Wolak & Finkelhor, 1998). Very little is known, however, about the percentage of children who become distressed and about what percentage are resilient to the exposure, or why. Furthermore, are the difficulties experienced by these children specifically caused by witnessing domestic violence or the cumulative effect of numerous family problems, such as parental alcoholism and divorce (e.g., Davies, Myers, Cummings, & Heindel, 1999)? Voluntary services aimed at increasing safety, ameliorating distress, and teaching healthier relationship skills are usually appropriate for children who witness violence.

Secondary Trauma

Secondary (or intergenerational) trauma occurs when a person, family, or community suffers trauma so extreme that it hinders their long-term ability to give care or otherwise fully participate in their family roles. Subsequently, even children and other relatives who were not exposed to the initial trauma may show signs that are similar to symptoms of posttraumatic stress, such as a generally restricted range of affect or "numbing," hyperarousal, and difficulty regulating emotional responses.

Secondary trauma is most closely associated with Holocaust survivors (Lev-Wiesel & Amir, 2001; Solomon, Kotler, & Mikulincer, 1988) and postcolonial American Indian communities (Duran, Duran, Woodis, & Woodis, 1998; Duran, Guillory, & Tingley, 1993) but can be relevant for any community that has suffered extreme violence or oppression in the present or recent past. Trauma and mourning for catastrophic losses in the past can produce lasting posttraumatic stress and depression in individuals that persist as they become spouses and parents. In many oppressed communities, in which virtually every member has experienced substantial trauma, there is the combined impact of what Richie (1997), in her analysis of partner violence in the African American community, called "intersecting oppressions." Research in secondary trauma has shown that trauma symptoms can manifest in spouses or children who did not experience the initial trauma through their contact with a seriously traumatized individual (Lev-Wiesel & Amir, 2001; Soloman et al., 1988). When working with individuals who belong to groups who have suffered secondary trauma, psychologists need to address the impact of that trauma as well as any recent or ongoing exposure (Duran et al., 1998).

CONCLUSION

Violence can affect any member of a family. The sequelae of violent victimization—which can include both the direct effects of assaults and the long-term effects of stress on a variety of bodily systems—are commonly seen in health care settings. All health care providers should have a basic knowledge of issues relevant to the spectrum of family violence victimization. Although each form of family violence has unique characteristics and specially tailored interventions, there are many commonalties among the various forms of violence in regard to dynamics, health consequences, and intervention. Understanding the similarities and differences across forms of violence can be a useful and productive means of establishing procedures to assess and intervene with victims of violence in health care settings.

REFERENCES

American Psychiatric Association. (1994). *Diagnostic and statistical manual of mental disorders* (4th ed.). Washington, DC: Author.

Anderson, C. M., Teicher, M. H., Polcari, A., & Renshaw, P. F. (2002). Abnormal T2 relaxation time in the cerebellar vermis of adults sexually abused in childhood: Potential role of the vermis in stress-enhanced risk for drug abuse. *Psychoneuroendocrinology, 27,* 231–244.

Banyard, V. L., & Hamby, S. L. (1996, August). *The experience of powerlessness and consequences of child sexual abuse.* Paper presented at the 104th Annual Convention of the American Psychological Association, Toronto, Ontario, Canada.

Berenson, A. B., Wiemann, C. M., Wilkinson, G. S., Jones, W. A., & Anderson, G. D. (1994). Perinatal morbidity associated with violence experienced by pregnant women. *American Journal of Obstetrics and Gynecology, 170,* 1760–1766.

Bolen, R. M., & Scannapieco, M. (1999, July). *Estimating the prevalence of child sexual abuse in North America.* Paper presented at the 6th International Family Violence Research Conference, Durham, NH.

Browne, A., & Finkelhor, D. (1986). Impact of child sexual abuse: A review of the research. *Psychological Bulletin, 99,* 66–77.

Connolly, A. M., Katz, V. L., Bash, K. L., McMahon, M. J., & Hansen, W. F. (1997). Trauma and pregnancy. *American Journal of Perinatology, 14,* 331–336.

Davies, P. T., Myers, R. L., Cummings, E. M., & Heindel, S. (1999). Adult conflict history and children's subsequent responses to conflict: An experimental test. *Journal of Family Psychology, 13,* 610–628.

Duran, E., Duran, B., Woodis, W., & Woodis, P. (1998). A postcolonial perspective on domestic violence in Indian country. In R. Carillo & J. Tello (Eds.), *Family violence and men of color: Healing the wounded male spirit* (pp. 95–113). New York: Springer.

Duran, E., Guillory, B., & Tingley, P. (1993). *Domestic violence in Native American communities: The effects of intergenerational posttraumatic stress.* Unpublished manuscript.

Edleson, J. L. (1999). The overlap between child maltreatment and woman battering. *Violence Against Women, 5*, 134–154.

Edleson, J. L. (in press). Should childhood exposure to adult domestic violence be defined as child maltreatment under the law? In P. G. Jaffe, L. L. Baker, & A. Cunningham (Eds.), *Ending domestic violence in the lives of children and parents: Promising practices for safety, healing, and prevention*. Toronto, Ontario, Canada: University of Toronto.

Fox, G. L., & Murry, V. M. (2000). Gender and families: Feminist perspectives and family research. *Journal of Marriage and the Family, 62*, 1160–1172.

Gazmararian, J. A., Lazorick, S., Spitz, A. M., Ballard, T. J., Saltzman, L. E., & Marks, J. S. (1996). Prevalence of violence against pregnant women. *Journal of the American Medical Association, 275*, 1915–1920.

Goodman, L. A., Koss, M. P., & Russo, N. F. (1993). Violence against women: Physical and mental health effects: Part 1. Research findings. *Applied and Preventive Psychology, 2*, 79–89.

Hamby, S. L. (1998). Partner violence: Prevention and intervention. In J. L. Jasinski & L. W. Williams (Eds.), *Partner violence: A comprehensive review of 20 years of research* (pp. 210–258). Thousand Oaks, CA: Sage.

Hamby, S. L., & Finkelhor, D. (1999). *The comprehensive juvenile victimization questionnaire*. Paper presented at Victimization of Children & Youth: An International Research Conference, Durham, NH.

Hamby, S. L., & Finkelhor, D. (2000). The victimization of children: Recommendations for assessment and instrument development. *Journal of the American Academy of Child and Adolescent Psychiatry, 39*, 829–840.

Hamby, S. L., & Finkelhor, D. (2001). *A guide to choosing and using questionnaires to measure the victimization of children* (Publication No. 186027). Washington, DC: Office of Juvenile Justice and Delinquency Prevention.

Hamby, S. L., & Koss, M. P. (2003). Violence against women: Risk factors, consequences and prevalence. In J. Liebschutz, S. Frayne, & G. Saxe (Eds.), *Violence against women: A physician's guide to identification and management* (pp. 3–38). Philadelphia: American College of Physicians–American Society of Internal Medicine Press.

Holmes, M. M., Resnick, H. S., Kilpatrick, D. G., & Best, C. L. (1996). Rape-related pregnancy: Estimates and descriptive characteristics from a national sample of women. *American Journal of Obstetrics and Gynecology, 175*, 320–325.

Kaufman Kantor, G., & Jasinski, J. L. (1998). Dynamics and risk factors in partner violence. In J. L. Jasinski & L. W. Williams (Eds.), *Partner violence: A comprehensive review of 20 years of research* (pp. 1–43). Thousand Oaks, CA: Sage.

Kendall-Tackett, K. A., & Eckenrode, J. (1997). The effects of neglect on academic achievement and disciplinary problems. In G. Kaufman Kantor & J. L. Jasinski (Eds.), *Out of the darkness: Contemporary perspectives on family violence* (pp. 105–112). Thousand Oaks, CA: Sage.

Kimerling, R., & Calhoun, K. S. (1994). Somatic symptoms, social support, and treatment seeking among sexual assault victims. *Journal of Consulting and Clinical Psychology, 62,* 333–340.

Koss, M. P., & Dinero, T. E. (1989). Discriminant analysis of risk factors for sexual victimization among a national sample of college women. *Journal of Consulting and Clinical Psychology, 57,* 242–250.

Koss, M. P., Ingram, M., & Pepper, S. (1997). Psychotherapists' role in the medical response to male partner violence. *Psychotherapy, 34,* 386–396.

Kropp, P. R., Hart, S. D., Webster, C. D., & Eaves, D. (1995). *Manual for the Spousal Assault Risk Assessment Guide* (2nd ed.). Vancouver, British Columbia, Canada: British Columbia Institute on Family Violence.

Lev-Wiesel, R., & Amir, M. (2001). Secondary traumatic stress, psychological distress, sharing of traumatic reminiscences, and marital quality among spouses of Holocaust child survivors. *Journal of Marital and Family Therapy, 27,* 433–444.

Mahoney, P., & Williams, L. W. (1998). Sexual assault in marriage: Prevalence, consequences, and treatment of wife rape. In J. L. Jasinski & L. W. Williams (Eds.), *Partner violence: A comprehensive review of 20 years of research* (pp. 113–162). Thousand Oaks, CA: Sage.

McFarlane, J., Parker, B., Soeken, K., & Bullock, L. (1992). Assessing for abuse during pregnancy: Severity and frequency of injuries and associated entry into prenatal care. *Journal of the American Medical Association, 267,* 3176–3178.

McLeer, S. V., & Anwar, R. (1989). A study of battered women presenting in an emergency department. *American Journal of Public Health, 79,* 65–66.

National Center for Health Statistics. (1994). *National Health and Nutrition Survey data tables.* Hyattsville, MD: Author.

National Center on Elder Abuse. (1998). *The national elder abuse incidence study.* Washington, DC: Author.

Parker, B., McFarlane, J., & Soeken, K. (1994). Abuse during pregnancy: Effects on maternal complications and birth weight in adult and teenage women. *Obstetrics and Gynecology, 84,* 323–328.

Pence, E. L. (1999). Some thoughts on philosophy. In M. F. Shepard & E. L. Pence (Eds.), *Coordinating community responses to domestic violence: Lessons from Duluth and beyond* (pp. 25–40). Thousand Oaks, CA: Sage.

Powers, S. K., & Howley, E. T. (1997). *Exercise physiology: Theory and application to fitness and performance* (3rd ed.). Dubuque, IA: Brown & Benchmark.

Raphael, J. (1999). The family violence option: An early assessment. *Violence Against Women, 5,* 449–466.

Richie, B. E. (1997, July). *Gender violence, racism, and social marginalization: Exploring the intersecting oppressions.* Paper presented at the 5th International Family Violence Research Conference, Durham, NH.

Schei, B., Samuelson, S. O., & Bakketeig, L. S. (1991). Does spousal physical abuse affect the outcome of pregnancy? *Scandinavian Journal of Social Medicine*, *19*, 26–31.

Shepard, M. F., & Pence, E. L. (Eds.). (1999). *Coordinating community responses to domestic violence: Lessons from Duluth and beyond*. Thousand Oaks, CA: Sage.

Shumway, J., O'Campo, P., Gielen, A., Witter, F. R., Khouzami, A. N., & Blakemore, K. J. (1999). Preterm labor, placental abruption, and premature rupture of membranes in relation to maternal violence or abuse. *Journal of Maternal Fetal Medicine*, *8*, 76–80.

Solomon, Z., Kotler, M., & Mikulincer, M. (1988). Combat-related posttraumatic stress disorder among second-generation Holocaust survivors: Preliminary findings. *American Journal of Psychiatry*, *145*, 865–868.

Stanko, E. A. (1988). Fear of crime and the myth of the safe home: A feminist critique of criminology. In K. Yllo & M. Bograd (Eds.), *Feminist perspectives on wife abuse* (pp. 75–88). Newbury Park, CA: Sage.

Stets, J. E., & Straus, M. A. (1990). Gender differences in reporting marital violence and its medical and psychological consequences. In M. A. Straus & R. J. Gelles (Eds.), *Physical violence in American families: Risk factors and adaptations to violence in 8,145 families* (pp. 151–165). New Brunswick, NJ: Transaction.

Straus, M. A., Hamby, S. L., Boney-McCoy, S., & Sugarman, D. B. (1996). The Revised Conflict Tactics Scales (CTS2): Development and preliminary psychometric data. *Journal of Family Issues*, *17*, 283–316.

Tjaden, P., & Thoennes, N. (2000). *Extent, nature, and consequences of intimate partner violence: Findings from the National Violence Against Women Survey*. Washington, DC: National Institutes of Justice.

Trocme, N., MacLaurin, B., Fallon, B., Daciuk , J., Billingsley, D., Tourigny, M., et al. (2001). *Canadian incidence study of reported child abuse and neglect*. Retrieved February 14, 2002, from http://www.hc-sc.gc.ca/hpb/lcdc/publicat/cisfr-ecirf/index.html

U.S. Bureau of the Census. (2001, October 5). *Historical income tables—People*. Retrieved February 13, 2002, from http://www.census.gov/hhes/histinc/p38a.html

Wolak, J., & Finkelhor, D. (1998). Children exposed to partner violence. In J. L. Jasinski & L. W. Williams (Eds.), *Partner violence: A comprehensive review of 20 years of research* (pp. 113–162). Thousand Oaks, CA: Sage.

I

INITIAL PRESENTATION OF FAMILY VIOLENCE IN HEALTH CARE SETTINGS

INTRODUCTION: INITIAL PRESENTATION OF FAMILY VIOLENCE IN HEALTH CARE SETTINGS

Family violence has many faces, and can present itself in a variety of ways. In this section, the authors describe various entry points into the health care system for people suffering from the effects of family violence. There is an overlap between the types of family violence that people experience, and the chapters in this section reflect that fact. However, each chapter has a primary focus of one specific type.

The first three chapters are concerned with domestic or intimate partner violence (IPV). Women in violent relationships are more likely to have surgery, as Chapter 2 describes. And this is why many enter the health care system. In Chapter 3, we learn of the unique issues faced by women of color who are in violent relationships, and how they might arise in health care settings. Chapter 4 describes how health care providers are often unwilling to intervene in these situations, even when obvious, due to institutional or personal factors. Although the primary focus is domestic violence, this chapter has relevance for all forms of family violence.

The next two chapters focus on child maltreatment. People who have suffered from abuse and other forms of childhood adversity are more prone to a wide range of chronic conditions as an adult, as chapter 5 describes. These patients are also high utilizers of health care services, giving providers many opportunities to screen for past and current abuse. In chapter 6, the needs of a specific population at risk for child maltreatment is highlighted—children with disabilities. As children, and later as adults, these people are often in contact with health care providers. Knowing that this is a high-risk population should encourage diligent screening on the part of health care providers.

The final two chapters in this section focus on the needs of older adults. Chapter 7 describes the physical and psychological symptoms that may indicate current elder abuse. Chapter 8 describes the normal developmental milestones of middle- and old age, and how adult survivors of childhood abuse might experience these. As adult survivors reach these milestones, they may manifest physical symptoms, which offer an opportunity for screening for past abuse.

All of these chapters will sensitize health care providers from a variety of fields to the many ways family violence can present in a health care setting.

2

SCREENING FOR FAMILY VIOLENCE WITH PERIOPERATIVE PATIENTS

DEBRA PILLING HASTINGS AND GLENDA KAUFMAN KANTOR

The surgical setting is one in which health care providers can screen for family violence. Abuse survivors have more lifetime surgeries than the general population, and many aspects of the surgical experience can trigger reactions that indicate past or current abuse. Mental health practitioners may be brought into perioperative settings to help patients who seem unusually anxious or frightened. They can also help patients who are facing surgery understand what to expect and how to cope. This chapter highlights some of the aspects of surgery that can be traumatizing for all types of abuse survivors and offers suggestions on how to screen for current intimate partner violence.

Ruth, a 20-year-old married woman, has been scheduled for exploratory surgery. She is to undergo a laparoscopy at her local community hospital in 2 weeks. Ruth has been experiencing abdominal discomfort, nausea, and vomiting off and on for several months. On occasion, she has noticed some vaginal bleeding. However, even after a complete history and physical, no definitive diagnosis could explain the reason for Ruth's symptoms. The surgeon knows Ruth's husband, having grown up in the same town with him. The husband seems quite supportive of Ruth and even accompanied her to this appointment. The surgeon decided to conduct exploratory surgery to further investigate the source of Ruth's discomfort and symptoms.

Two weeks later, in preparation for the surgery, nurses performed their preoperative assessment of Ruth. They inquired about her height, weight, allergies to drugs, and history of smoking. They asked if she might be pregnant. The nurses measured Ruth's temperature, pulse, and blood pressure. They assumed that her husband, who had accompanied his wife to the hospital, would be a strong source of support for her after discharge.

SCREENING FOR FAMILY VIOLENCE IN PERIOPERATIVE SETTINGS

The above vignette illustrates two missed opportunities for screening for family violence. It is unfortunate that while gathering information from Ruth, the surgeon did not ask about the status of her current relationship with her partner. Similarly, during the assessment on the morning of surgery, the nurse never asked Ruth about the presence of domestic violence in her life. If the health care practitioners had asked, a possible explanation for Ruth's physical problems may have been discovered, and the preoperative nursing assessment might have identified a need for several additional interventions.

It is normal to be anxious or fearful when faced with impending surgery. Most people fear not knowing what to expect, what the experience will be like, or what the outcome may be. Women who have experienced interpersonal violence often have additional concerns. For example, someone who has been abused may have a strong reaction to being physically held or strapped down with a safety belt on the operating room bed—a routine occurrence in the surgical suite. Similarly, a procedure that requires a woman to be placed in a lithotomy position or "stirrups"—an intraoperative position required for a number of surgical procedures—may create anxiety in women who have experienced sexual victimization such as vaginal or anal penetration. Memory of past experiences—long hidden, or buried—may resurface. Survivors may also experience distrust of individuals in unfamiliar surroundings, such as in an operating room. Fear of experiencing a loss of control or the inability to take care of oneself while in this environment may be evident. The use of anesthetic or pain medications may cause concern for a woman who is anxious about a diminished level of awareness. She may fear a perceived inability to protect her physical being. The presence of these concerns could indicate past or current abuse.

Ruth's story unfortunately mirrors that of many abused women who confront the health care system on a daily basis. Most women do not volunteer a history of abuse when seeing their health care providers, and many health professionals—including therapists—do not consistently ask (Aldarondo & Straus, 1994; McCauley et al., 1995).

Most of the recent research on the need for screening in health care settings is focused on women who have been battered by an intimate partner. However, as other chapters in this volume indicate, abusive histories can encompass a wide variety of traumatic events, including neglect, sexual molestation, rape, and psychological and physical abuse. Victimizations can be singular events, or they can be ongoing. The impact of traumatic events will also vary depending on a number of factors, such as the age of onset, chronicity of abuse, the individual's relationship to the perpetrator, individual attributes, and characteristics of the broader environment in which the abuse occurred. One thing, however, is known: Women with a past or current history of abuse have surgery significantly more often than their nonabused counterparts.

In this chapter we review the literature on the relationship of women's victimization histories to surgical intervention, because it is an important entry point into the health care system. Medical personnel should be alert to symptoms that can indicate the presence of abuse. Mental health practitioners can also screen for abuse and can help abuse survivors cope with the challenges they face when they prepare for surgery. We present a theoretical framework for guiding the screening and assisting of abused patients who might be facing surgery. Finally, we address implications for practice.

LIFETIME ABUSE AND ADULT HEALTH OUTCOMES

Intimate partner violence (IPV) is now generally recognized as a significant health problem and is believed by many to have reached widespread proportions in the United States (Aldarondo & Straus, 1994; Bullock & Schornstein, 1998; Jasinski & Kaufman Kantor, 2001). Intimate partner violence is responsible for an estimated one quarter to one half of all women presenting for treatment in emergency rooms (U.S. Department of Justice, 1998); it may be part of a system of domination and control that includes emotional, verbal, and economic abuse and sexual assault, coercion, or injury (Kaufman Kantor & Jasinski, 1998).

Because of the saliency and severity of the acute trauma experienced by some victims of IPV, studies have focused on victims who are seen in acute-care settings. Facial lacerations and skull, neck, and orbital trauma can occur as a result of direct force or assault to the head, neck, and face (Hartzell, Botek, & Goldbert, 1996; Ochs, Neuenschwander, & Dodson, 1996). Various types of fractures have been documented in women either from direct force or from the victims' attempts to defend themselves. Internal injuries to the spleen, liver, and kidney occur when patients are punched or kicked in the abdomen or back. In addition, forced sexual intercourse can cause vaginal bleeding, vaginal or anal tearing, or hemorrhoids. Many of these conditions require surgical intervention. Berrios and Grady (1991) reviewed data from 218 women who self-identified as victims of IPV at an emergency department in the San Francisco Bay area and found that over one quarter of these victims were admitted to the hospital for their index injury and that 13% required major surgical treatment.

Childhood abuse can also set the stage for symptoms that lead to surgery in adults. For example, a history of childhood victimization was significantly associated with physical symptoms such as nausea, diarrhea, constipation, fatigue, insomnia, abdominal pain, back pain, soft-tissue pain, chest pain, and multiple hospital admissions for undefined conditions (Bullock & Schornstein, 1998; Drossman et al., 1990; Eby, Campbell, Sullivan, & Davidson, 1995; Walker et al., 1999).

Past abuse can lead to current abuse. Female survivors of childhood sexual abuse are also at higher risk of sexual revictimization as adults (Grauerholz, 2000). West, Williams, and Siegel (2000) compared women who had been sexually abused in childhood only to women who were victimized as both children and adults. They found that women who were revictimized were more likely to experience infertility, repeated vaginal infections, sexually transmitted diseases, and painful intercourse. Surgery may be suggested to aid in the treatment of these symptoms.

Women's Victimization History and Surgical Intervention

Studies of women seeking care from gastroenterology services also point to a link between victimization histories and surgery. In their study of 206 women seeking care in a gastroenterology practice, Drossman et al. (1990) found that female patients who had experienced abuse as either an adult or a child had more surgeries over the course of a lifetime than did the patients who had not experienced abuse. Among female patients seen for medical problems, a history of abuse was associated with more pelvic and abdominal pain and more surgeries over their lifetimes. Similarly, Leserman et al. (1996), in their interviews with 239 women seeking care at a gastroenterology clinic, found that women with a history of physical and sexual abuse (66.5%) experienced more surgeries than those who had not been abused.

We analyzed intake data from a matched sample of 53 nonabused and 57 abused female patients drawn from a primary-care practice in northern New England (Kendall-Tackett, Marshall, & Ness, 2000) and found that women who had experienced IPV in adulthood were twice as likely to undergo major surgery as women who identified no abuse (Hastings & Kaufman Kantor, 2003). In addition, the results showed that the outcomes of women's victimization included significantly more major surgical interventions, especially surgery of an exploratory nature. Earlier assessment of abuse may have led to more conservative interventions that precluded a need for exploratory surgery (Hastings & Kaufman Kantor, 2003).

The findings of our study provide support for the stress–illness perspective we used to frame the analysis and were consistent with previous research correlating women's victimization experiences with health impairment. The analyses showed that women with a self-reported history of abuse also experienced significantly more symptoms of depression and fatigue than their nonabused counterparts. We concluded that the combination of experiencing childhood abuse and IPV places women at an even higher risk for multiple symptoms, especially depression. Although few women reported suicidal thoughts, such thoughts were more likely when women experienced multiple victimizations across the life course. Comparisons of women who had experienced abuse either as a child, as an adult, or both, supported the theory that cumulative victimization causes greater stress and more adverse effects (Hastings & Kaufman Kantor, 2003).

A history of victimization can also influence recovery from surgery. Wukasch (1996) studied the impact that a history of rape or incest (or both) had on women who were recovering from a specific type of surgical intervention: elective hysterectomies. In this cross-sectional study, 92 women were interviewed at four established times in the postsurgical period, each several months apart. The results showed a significantly higher level of depression in the first year after hysterectomy among women with a sexual assault history compared with nonvictimized women. Wukasch suggested that undergoing a hysterectomy could trigger past traumatic memories of abuse. Depression might result when the victim is forced to deal not only with the surgical experience but also with the renewed memory of the abuse. There is no indication that Wukasch measured current abuse.

Victimization History and Psychological Symptoms

Anxiety, depression (Sutherland, Bybee, & Sullivan, 1998), posttraumatic stress disorder (PTSD; Silva, McFarlane, Soeken, Parker, & Reel, 1997), somatization, low self-esteem, and suicidal ideation (McCauley et al., 1995) are well documented in the literature as symptoms that women who have been physically, sexually, or emotionally abused in intimate relationships or in childhood are known to experience. Studies of abused women in a variety of contexts, such as primary-care settings (Silva et al., 1997), psychiatric facilities (Farley & Keaney, 1997), drug treatment facilities (Gil-Rivas, Fiorentine, & Anglin, 1996), and domestic violence shelters (Astin, Lawrence, & Foy, 1993; Street & Arias, 2001) have documented the prevalence and severity of PTSD.

Abused women have characteristics similar to those of other traumatized populations and are more likely to manifest symptoms of PTSD when the levels of physical and verbal abuse are high, when threat is perceived, and when they have been victims of forced sex (Kemp, Green, Hovanitz, & Rawlings, 1995). Several studies support findings that the incidence of PTSD is particularly high among survivors of child sexual abuse (e.g., Messman-Moore, Long, & Siegfried, 2000). Silva et al. (1997) recommended that clinicians ask abused women about dreams, flashbacks, or terror attacks related to abuse to assess for further symptoms of PTSD.

Anxiety is believed by many health care practitioners to be a common stressor in dealing with the prospect of impending surgery. Calvin and Lane's (1999) study of male and female orthopedic patients found that all of these patients experienced some preoperative uncertainty and anxiety, regardless of the acuity level of the diagnosis or pending surgery. Wiens (1998) specifically examined preoperative anxiety and fear in women. She found that each woman in her study experienced the upcoming surgery in her own individual way and that the uniqueness of the event was related to previous and current personal life experiences. She suggested that the setting in which preoperative care takes place should be one in which women feel comfortable communicating their fears about the impending surgery. Often the anxieties that women are experiencing may be related not directly to the surgery, as one might assume, but rather to past or present personal life events. For women with histories of abuse, sensitivity in communication is essential to provide them an opportunity to verbalize their unique fears and anxieties. This disclosure can be facilitated by both medical and mental health practitioners.

Stress and anxiety may also affect recovery from surgery by means of their effects on immune competency and wound healing (e.g., Kiecolt-Glaser, Page, Marucha, MacCallum, & Glaser, 1998). Emotions have a direct effect on stress hormones that in turn affect the function of the immune system. Suppressed immune function could result in poorer surgical outcomes. Women who have a history of victimization—particularly those who are enduring violence in current relationships—may be at higher risk for such postoperative complications given the presence of this particular stressor in their lives. This is just one area in which clinicians might facilitate more positive outcomes for their patients.

THEORETICAL FRAMEWORK FOR INTERVENTION

There are no specific studies to guide professionals as to which interventions are best for assisting abused individuals who are facing surgery. However, there is long-standing theoretical and empirical support for a stress–illness linkage (Dohrenwend & Dohrenwend, 1974; Turner & Lloyd, 1995) that suggests this model as an appropriate framework for intervention. For the most part, research has looked at the association among social stress, life stress, and outcomes related to emotional health and well-being. Adversity and victimization across the life span also are associated with psychological distress and physical illness (Barr, Boyce, & Zeltzer, 1996; Giles-Sims, 1998; Leserman et al., 1996). The actual physiological mechanism underlying victimization–illness associations has not typically been examined by researchers in the field of IPV.

Drawing on a body of neuroscience research (e.g., Schwarz & Perry, 1994), Kendall-Tackett (2000) speculated on the causal paths that link childhood victimization with chronic illness experienced by adults. For example, the findings of higher levels of depression and PTSD are well established among adults who experienced abuse as children. People who have experienced significant trauma in their lives are more vulnerable to the effects of subsequent stressors, a result of a state of chronic hyperarousal. This means that the body overreacts to subsequent new stressors by regularly producing excessive levels of stress hormones.

In the past, stress researchers may have underestimated the contributions of cumulative adversities to emotional distress (Turner & Lloyd, 1995). Further elaboration of the biological effects of stress linked to victimization experiences are seen in studies that have examined wound healing (Constantino, Sekula, Rabin, & Stone, 2000; Glaser et al., 1999); for example, Constantino and colleagues (2000) studied immune function in abused women and found lower T-cell function in the abused group. Glaser et al. (1999) investigated the effect of stress or fear on surgical outcomes such as wound healing. Citing research that psychological stress delays wound healing, they investigated 36 women and found that psychological stress can have marked adverse consequences for immunologic activity that must take place at wound sites for healing to occur. Circumstances that upset the balance of immunologic competence, such as stress, can impair the local inflammatory response. These findings are also consistent with the current psychosomatic medicine literature on the relevance of psychological influences to postoperative recuperation.

IMPLICATIONS FOR PRACTICE

Underlying the purpose of this chapter is a concern that female victims of IPV undergo surgical intervention without prior screening, identification, or appropriate assessment of the existence of violence in their lives. Similarly, when faced with impending surgery, are women who seek additional psychological support appropriately assessed and prepared? In today's fast-paced perioperative setting, with often minimal time spent in the hospital setting after surgery, are victimized women returning to the home environment in a vulnerable state without appropriate intervention or referral regarding ongoing abuse in their lives? The following are some specific suggestions for intervention with patients. The ultimate goal is to improve the care and support of patients who struggle with the memory of victimization or ongoing interpersonal violence in their lives. Medical and mental health professionals must support the practices that best address issues of IPV in patients who are facing impending surgery.

Screen for Past and Current Violence

Previous studies point to the need for comprehensive knowledge of the victimization and status of patients. A history of abuse should be identified through a routine, comprehensive screening on past and current victimization at all points of entry into the health care system (Aldarondo & Straus, 1994; Family Violence Prevention Fund, 1999). Aldarondo and Straus (1994) asserted that without direct inquiry, patients are unlikely to report violence in their lives. Screening is easily achieved by using standardized instruments such as the Conflict Tactics Scale (Straus, 1988) or by asking a direct question in a manner similar to the following: "Because I see so many women(/patients) in my practice who have experienced intimate violence in their past or in their relationship with a current partner, I now ask all my patients this question: Do you feel safe in your relationship with your partner?"

Often, a single screening question, asked in a safe environment, will prompt a patient to provide information about presence or history of abuse. If a patient responds affirmatively and is comfortable discussing the issue, further assessment might reveal the extent of the abuse and ways in which the patient has coped thus far.

If a victim chooses to not reveal history or presence of abuse, but its presence is still suspected, then there are classic signs or symptoms that alert one to IPV. Physical signs include the presence of any injury, particularly an injury that is unexplained or one for which the explanation does not match the severity. Evidence of bruises in various stages of healing, a delay in seeking care or treatment, or repeated visits to the clinician with vague complaints may also be indicative of an ongoing abusive relationship.

Other signs of possible IPV include drug or alcohol dependence or overdose, or stress-related physical or emotional complaints. Behavioral clues might include evasiveness on the part of the patient, an unwillingness to speak or share information in front of a partner, or presence of an overly controlling or "protective" partner. A clinician should also be alert when treating pregnant women and new mothers, because pregnancy does not provide immunity from abuse (Jasinski & Kaufman Kantor, 2001).

Gerbert, Abercrombie, Caspers, Lowe, and Bronstone (1999) suggested that clinicians who suspect ongoing abuse even after the patient denies its presence should proceed by reaffirming that abuse is wrong and acknowledging the patient's worth. As noted above, not all women are at a point where they are ready to disclose sensitive information about their lives when they enter a particular health care setting. They should not be forced to do so. A dilemma lies in the fact that without direct questioning, abuse may remain hidden, physical and psychological distress can go unabated, and appropriate interventions may not be delivered. However, it remains of utmost importance that women are free to disclose such information at a time and in a place with which they are comfortable. Disclosure is ultimately the woman's decision.

Provide Appropriate Support

Greater awareness and understanding of the lived experience of patients allow practitioners to provide more appropriate and supportive intervention. For example, verbal reinforcement to the patient that the abuse is not his or her fault is crucial. Many victims assume that they are at least in part responsible for what they have experienced at the hands of their loved one; this may have been stated repeatedly by the abusers themselves. It is crucial not only that clinicians inform patients that they are not to blame but also that they reinforce that the patient does not deserve this treatment and validate that he or she is worthy of and deserves better (Gerbert et al., 1999).

Increase Awareness Among Health Care Providers

Advocates for battered women and health care and mental health professionals are currently working nationwide to educate the public, especially health care providers, about IPV. This represents an effort to enhance the awareness of IPV as a health care issue for women and to provide optimum, and appropriate, health services to battered women seeking care and safety through contact with health professionals. This includes routine screening, assessment, intervention, and awareness of local or community resources, including local women's crisis centers. Professionals with the most training in domestic violence hold victims less responsible and are more willing to provide appropriate intervention (Rose & Saunders, 1986).

Optimal outcomes are most likely when clinicians view disclosure as a process whereby work at reprocessing past trauma should be balanced with the need for more immediate interventions (Aldarondo & Straus, 1994; Evans & Sullivan, 1995).

REFERENCES

Aldarondo, E., & Straus, M. A. (1994). Screening for physical violence in couple therapy: Methodological, practical, and ethical considerations. *Family Process, 33*, 425–439.

Astin, M. C., Lawrence, K. J., & Foy, D. W. (1993). Posttraumatic stress disorder among battered women: Risk and resiliency factors. *Violence and Victims, 8*, 17–28.

Barr, R. G., Boyce, W. T., & Zeltzer, L. K. (1996). The stress–illness association in children: A perspective from the biobehavioral interface. In R. J. Haggerty, L. R. Sherrod, N. Garmezy, & M. Rutter (Eds.), *Stress, risk, and resilience in children and adolescents: Processes, mechanisms, and interventions* (pp. 182–224). Cambridge, England: Cambridge University Press.

Berrios, D. C., & Grady, D. (1991). Domestic violence: Risk factors and outcomes. *Western Journal of Medicine, 155*, 133–135.

Bullock, K. A., & Schornstein, S. L. (1998). Improving medical care for victims of domestic violence. *Hospital Physician, 34*(9), 42–58.

Calvin, R. L., & Lane, P. L. (1999). Perioperative uncertainty and state anxiety of orthopaedic surgical patients. *Orthopaedic Nursing, 18*(6), 61–66.

Constantino, R. E., Sekula, L. K., Rabin, B., & Stone, C. (2000). Negative life experiences, depression, and immune function in abused and nonabused women. *Biological Research for Nursing, 1*, 190–198.

Dohrenwend, B. S., & Dohrenwend, B. P. (Eds.). (1974). *Stressful life events: Their nature and events.* New York: Wiley.

Drossman, D. A., Leserman, J., Nachman, G., Li, Z., Gluck, H., Toomey, T. C., & Mitchell, C. M. (1990). Sexual and physical abuse in women with functional or organic gastrointestinal disorders. *Annals of Internal Medicine, 113*, 828–833.

Eby, K. K., Campbell, J. C., Sullivan, C. M., & Davidson, W. S. (1995). Health effects of experiences of sexual violence for women with abusive partners. *Health Care for Women International, 16*, 563–576.

Evans, K., & Sullivan, J. M. (1995). *Treating addicted survivors of trauma.* New York: Guilford Press.

Family Violence Prevention Fund. (1999). *Preventing domestic violence: Clinical guidelines on routine screening.* Washington, DC: U.S. Department of Health and Human Services.

Farley, M., & Keaney, J. C. (1997). Physical symptoms, somatization, and dissociation in women survivors of childhood sexual assault. *Women and Health, 25*(3), 33–45.

Gerbert, B., Abercrombie, P., Caspers, N., Lowe, C., & Bronstone, A. (1999). How healthcare providers help battered women: The survivors' perspective. *Women and Health, 29*(3), 115–135.

Giles-Sims, J. (1998). The aftermath of partner violence. In J. L. Jasinski & L. M. Williams (Eds.), *Partner violence: A comprehensive review of 20 years of research* (pp. 44–72). Thousand Oaks, CA: Sage.

Gil-Rivas, V., Fiorentine, R., & Anglin, M. D. (1996). Sexual abuse, physical abuse, and posttraumatic stress disorder among women participating in outpatient drug abuse treatment. *Journal of Psychoactive Drugs, 28*, 95–102.

Glaser, R., Kiecolt-Glaser, J. K., Marucha, P. T., MacCallum, R. C., Laskowski, B. F., & Malarkey, W. B. (1999). Stress-related changes in proinflammatory cytokine production in wounds. *Archives of General Psychiatry, 56*, 450–456.

Grauerholz, L. (2000). An ecological approach to understanding sexual revictimization: Linking personal, interpersonal, and sociological factors and processes. *Child Maltreatment, 5*(1), 5–17.

Hartzell, K. N., Botek, A. A., & Goldbert, S. H. (1996). Orbital fractures in women due to sexual assault and domestic violence. *Ophthalmology, 103*, 953–957.

Hastings, D. P., & Kaufman Kantor, G. (2003). The relationship of women's victimization history to surgical intervention. *AORN Journal, 77*, 163–180.

Jasinski, J., & Kaufman Kantor, G. (2001). Pregnancy, stress and wife assault: Ethnic differences in prevalence, severity, and onset in a national sample. *Violence and Victims, 16*, 219–232.

Kaufman Kantor, G., & Jasinski, J. L. (1998). Dynamics and risk factors in partner violence. In J. L. Jasinski & L. M. Williams (Eds.), *Partner violence: A comprehensive review of 20 years of research* (pp. 1–43). Thousand Oaks, CA: Sage.

Kemp, A., Green, B. L., Hovanitz, C., & Rawlings, E. I. (1995). Incidence and correlates of posttraumatic stress disorder in battered women: Shelter and community samples. *Journal of Interpersonal Violence, 10*(1), 43–55.

Kendall-Tackett, K. A. (2000). Physiological correlates of child abuse: Chronic hyperarousal in PTSD, depression, and irritable bowel syndrome. *Child Abuse and Neglect, 24*, 799–810.

Kendall-Tackett, K. A., Marshall, R., & Ness, K. E. (2000). Victimization, health-care use, and health maintenance. *Family Violence and Sexual Assault Bulletin, 16*, 18–21.

Kiecolt-Glaser, J., Page, G. G., Marucha, P. T., MacCallum, R. C., & Glaser, R. (1998). Psychological influences on surgical recovery: Perspectives from psychoneuroimmunology. *American Psychologist, 53*, 1209–1218.

Leserman, J., Drossman, D. A., Li, Z., Toomey, T. C., Nachman, G., & Glogau, L. (1996). Sexual and physical abuse history in gastroenterology practice: How types of abuse impact health status. *Psychosomatic Medicine, 58*, 4–15.

McCauley, J., Kern, D. E., Kolodner, K., Dill, L., Schroeder, A. F., DeChant, H. K., et al. (1995). The "battering syndrome": Prevalence and clinical characteristics of domestic violence in primary care internal medicine practices. *Annals of Internal Medicine, 123*, 737–746.

Messman-Moore, T. L., Long, P. J., & Siegfried, N. J. (2000). The revictimization of child sexual abuse survivors: An examination of the adjustment of college women with child sexual abuse, adult sexual assault, and adult physical abuse. *Child Maltreatment, 5*(1), 18–27.

Ochs, H. A., Neuenschwander, M. C., & Dodson, T. B. (1996). Are head, neck and facial injuries markers of domestic violence? *Journal of the American Dental Association, 127*, 757–761.

Rose, K., & Saunders, D. G. (1986). Nurses' and physicians' attitudes about women abuse: The effects of gender and professional role. *Health Care for Women International, 7*, 427–438.

Schwarz, E. D., & Perry, B. D. (1994). The posttraumatic response in children and adolescents. *Psychiatric Clinics of North America, 17*, 311–326.

Silva, C., McFarlane, J., Soeken, K., Parker, B., & Reel, S. (1997). Symptoms of post-traumatic stress disorder in abused women in a primary care setting. *Journal of Women's Health, 6*, 543–552.

Straus, M. A. (1988). *Manual for the Conflict Tactics Scales (CTS)*. Family Research Laboratory, University of New Hampshire (Durham).

Street, A. E., & Arias, I. (2001). Psychological abuse and posttraumatic stress disorder in battered women: Explaining the roles of shame and guilt. *Violence and Victims, 16*, 65–78.

Sutherland, C., Bybee, D., & Sullivan, C. (1998). The long-term effects of battering on women's health. *Women's Health, 4*, 41–70.

Turner, R. J., & Lloyd, D. A. (1995). Lifetime traumas and mental health: The significance of cumulative adversity. *Journal of Health and Social Behavior, 36*, 360–376.

U.S. Department of Justice (1998). *Violence by inmates*. Washington, DC: BJS Clearinghouse.

Walker, E. A., Gelfand, A., Katon, W. J., Koss, M. P., Von Korff, M., Bernstein, D., & Russo, J. (1999). Adult health status of women with histories of childhood abuse and neglect. *American Journal of Medicine, 107*, 332–339.

West, C. M., Williams, L. M., & Siegel, J. A. (2000). Adult sexual revictimization among Black women sexually abused in childhood: A prospective examination of serious consequences of abuse. *Child Maltreatment, 5*, 49–57.

Wiens, A. G. (1998). Preoperative anxiety in women. *Association of Operating Room Nurses Journal, 68*, 74–88.

Wukasch, R. N. (1996). The impact of a history of rape and incest on the posthysterectomy experience. *Health Care for Women International, 17*, 47–55.

3

DOMESTIC VIOLENCE INTERVENTIONS WITH WOMEN OF COLOR: THE INTERSECTION OF VICTIMIZATION AND CULTURAL DIVERSITY

CATHERINE KOVEROLA AND SUBADRA PANCHANADESWARAN

The negative impact of partner violence on women's health has been well established. It also is known that ethnic minority women are often in poorer health than their White counterparts. What happens when minority status and partner violence intersect? All women in battering relationships face barriers to leaving these relationships and living their lives free from violence. These barriers are compounded for women of color. Poverty, language barriers, illegal immigration status, and racism all limit their options. The longer they are in these relationships, the greater the negative impact on their physical and mental health. This chapter offers an exploratory glimpse into the lives of battered women of color and how their culture shapes their ability to leave and their willingness to seek help.

Domestic violence between adult partners cuts across all social classes, ethnic groups, cultures, and age groups (Hall & Lynch, 1998). In the United States, changing demographics and immigration policies (McGee, 1997) have significantly affected the U.S. ethnic composition; the nation now comprises diverse populations and varied cultures. Despite the universality of the phenomenon of violence against women, a community's experiences of migration, racism, history of colonization, religious beliefs, and socialization norms affect the patterns of interpersonal violence experienced by women in ethnic communities (Almeida & Durkin, 1999), making their responses group specific (Barnes, 1999, p. 357). In a recent report on the impact of culture, race, and ethnicity, Surgeon General David Satcher noted the following:

> The cultures from which people hail affect all aspects of mental health and illness, including the types of stresses they confront, whether they seek help, what types of help they seek, what symptoms and concerns they bring to clinical attention, and what types of coping styles and social supports they possess. (U.S. Department of Health and Human Services, 2001, p. 10)

Racial and cultural differences are also important factors that affect abused women's help-seeking behavior as well as the interventions targeted for them.

Feminist movements, theorists, and treatment models to end violence against women have been criticized for their "Eurocentricism" in that they are perceived to exclude the perspectives of women of color (Kanuha, 1994, p. 429). Disadvantaged women of color, who typically have low levels of resources and support, experience heightened vulnerability in the face of their inability to deal with intimate partner violence (Thompson et al., 2000). Hence, it has been increasingly recognized that it is vital to place abused women's experiences in the context of their cultural beliefs and their racial experiences. In addition, an understanding of the honor systems prevalent in certain communities can help practitioners understand the phenomenon of female homicide and intervene effectively (Baker, 1999).

HEALTH CONSEQUENCES OF ABUSE

What are the health effects of domestic violence for women of color? Our most conservative estimate is that they are similar to those of White women. Most abuse survivors suffer significant long-term physical, emotional, psychological, and behavioral problems, as described in previous research (Bohn & Holz, 1996). However, these effects are most likely compounded by the negative impact of racism, poverty, and discrimination. Racial and ethnic disparities in health are common, and the disparities in mental health are even greater than those in physical health. Indeed, individuals at the lowest strata of income, education, and occupation are two to three times more likely to have a mental disorder than people at higher socioeconomic strata. Ethnic minorities in general are overrepresented in the lowest strata, and conditions such as depression can have a profound impact on health (U.S. Department of Health and Human Services, 2001).

Women of color who are subjected to abuse by intimate partners could experience a higher degree of adverse consequences because of the multitude of issues that hinder rightful acknowledgment of abuse experiences and appropriate and timely help seeking. Some preliminary research has revealed health effects that are more severe for women of color in battering relationships. For example, Thompson et al. (2000) found that abused African American women not only experienced higher psychological distress but also perceived themselves as having significantly lower levels of social support. In another study, psychological abuse was positively correlated with yeast infections, depression, and hypertension among abused Black women (Lawson, Rodgers-Rose, & Rajaram, 1999).

In Acevedo's (2000) qualitative study, Mexican American women had been severely battered, leading to vision impairment; punched in the stomach, leading to hospitalization; choked, and whipped with a butcher's knife. However, some of the participants were unwilling to label their experiences as abuse and used their cultural values of tolerance and need to preserve their families to explain their experiences. Degree of acculturation also determines the extent to which minority women would view their abusive experiences or seek help, especially among Latina women (Mattson & Rodriguez, 1999).

The Surgeon General's report recommended integration of mental health services into primary care because this is often more acceptable to minorities seeking mental health services. Screening for abuse can be part of the mental health services provided, but it must be done in such a way that the women's culture is respected. Lack of cultural competence may deter women of color from seeking services at all (U.S. Department of Health and Human Services, 2001).

BARRIERS FACED BY WOMEN OF COLOR

How does a woman of color who is a victim of domestic violence present to the professional? Most often, she does not present at all. She does not call to schedule an appointment. She lives in isolation and fear, unable to reach out for help. When developing services for battered women of color, it is important to think outside of the traditional scope of service delivery, in a clinic or private practice. Although some women do voluntarily present for services in a mental health setting, the vast majority do not. Referrals may include a mother who is court-ordered for treatment on the threat of losing her children to child protective services; a woman referred from an emergency department subsequent to treatment for acute violence-related injuries; a woman referred by a family practice physician who senses something is amiss but is not sure what; or a woman from a domestic violence shelter. The majority of women, however, will not be referred. These are women restricted to the confines of their own homes, which have become virtual prisons.

Other chapters in this book highlight the multitude of barriers faced by victims of family violence in their effort to seek help, obtain help, and embrace a violence-free life. The barriers for a woman of color are even more numerous and often seem to be insurmountable. These barriers include language; traditional beliefs; cultural norms; religion; fear of legal consequences, such as deportation and loss of children; and fear of discrimination and racism.

Culture is the cumulative transmission of social norms, practices, religious beliefs, language, and art across generations (Almeida & Durkin, 1999). Changing cultural norms invariably affect perpetrators, survivors, and advocates against domestic violence. Often, cultural beliefs of minority groups are minimized or misunderstood by the dominant community domestic violence practitioners (Almeida & Dolan-Delvecchio, 1999). To truly be part of a healing process with women of color who are victims of domestic violence, professionals must acquire additional knowledge and skills to become culturally competent. Most important of all, however, the clinician must always be willing to humbly ask "Is there anything you can tell me about your culture or community that will help me to understand your health better, so that I can be most helpful to you?" (Pinn & Chunko, 1997).

Although extensive research on abused women has been conducted in recent years, little attention has been paid to battered women among immigrant communities and ethnic minority groups (Bui & Morash, 1999; Mattson & Rodriguez, 1999). Women from immigrant communities face multiple stressors in terms of adjustments and transitions, under- or unemployment and resulting economic hardships, low levels of education and skill, and the changes in role prescriptions that make them vulnerable to abuse from their partners (Firestone, Lambert, & Vega, 1999; Segal, 2000). In an immigrant family's new environment, exposure to ideals and social norms different from their own cultural values create further stress. Furthermore, language barriers and fear of deportation pose real hurdles for immigrant women. Because of all these factors, women's vulnerability is significantly heightened. Even with a high degree of acculturation, women often resort to traditional methods of coping when faced with abusive situations (Mattson & Rodriguez, 1999).

In the following composite case examples, the experiences of three women highlight the barriers faced by abused women of color endeavoring to embrace a violence-free life. Their experiences underscore the importance of culturally competent professionals who were able to effectively intervene.

MARIA

At age 16, I came to the U.S. from Mexico. My parents had heard of a better life in the U.S., and they gave their life savings to the Coyote to bring me here. On the journey, I was raped repeatedly every night, as were most of the young girls. I became pregnant. Jose took me as his wife, and for three years he beat me daily. One day he left me, penniless and with two small children. I spoke little English and had few friends. But determined to survive, I looked for work in the factories of Los Angeles. A nearby mission took care of my children while I worked.

In the factory, I met John. He was an American, and he treated me well at first. For the first time since leaving Mexico I felt loved. My babies had food, clothes, and a place to sleep. I was able to send money to my family. We had a wedding; this was the best day of my life. The dream my parents had for me had come true. Happiness, however, lasted only until I became pregnant. Then the abuse began. It all blurs, just as with Jose. I was too ashamed to tell my parents in my letters. They had become so proud of me. Many times I went to the hospital with serious injuries from the beatings. One of the times that I was very badly hurt, my husband brought me to the hospital. He was quite frightened by my injuries. I recall that visit very clearly. A nurse asked him to leave my bedside, and then in Spanish she quietly began to ask me about my injuries, asking how I had sustained them. I told her that I had fallen down the stairs. She said "a lot of women with injuries like yours have been hurt by someone they love." And "that usually the person is afraid to tell. Afraid something bad will happen." She asked me what I was afraid of. I was so afraid. I began to cry. She asked if I was afraid of the legal repercussions. I explained that my husband said that if I told anyone he would call the INS (Immigration and Naturalization Services), and I would have to leave the country and that he would keep all my babies. She began to tell me about a new law, the Violence Against Women (VAW) act, that would provide me with the possibility of gaining legal status. I began to have a glimmer of hope.

CLINICAL DIRECTIVES

Maria's road to healing began with the intervention of a Spanish-speaking medical practitioner who used the JCAHO-recommended (Joint Commission for the Accreditation of Healthcare Organizations) screening questions (Feldhaus et al., 1997; Shea, Mahoney, & Lacey, 1997). Countless women who seek health care, both acute and routine, are never screened for domestic violence, even when they present with classic domestic violence injury patterns (Bohn & Holz, 1996; Campbell, Pliska, Taylor, & Sheridan, 1994; Fanslow, Norton, & Spinola, 1998). This particular health care practitioner followed the recommended protocol of screening in private and in the native language of the patient.

It is very important to not screen in front of the perpetrator, who often accompanies the victim to the medical facility. This seems like an obvious error; however, it is an error that is sadly made often for practical reasons. The perpetrator may be the only one who speaks English, while the victim does not (Pinn & Chunko, 1997; Shea et al., 1997). It is also important not to have children function in the role of interpreter. Children of immigrant parents are often thrust in the role of translator–interpreter, so again, this often occurs naturally. However, in the situation of domestic violence, it places the child at risk. The perpetrator may subsequently interrogate the child, who may unwittingly disclose information that can compromise the safety of both mother and children. It also places the child in an inappropriate role within the family (Koverola & Morahan, 2001; Zink, 2000).

It is vital to provide undocumented women information about the VAW Act. The passage of the VAW Act provided a route of freedom for scores of undocumented women living in the United States. In brief, the law essentially permits an undocumented woman who is married to a U.S. citizen or legal resident, who is a victim of domestic violence, and who chooses to proceed with a divorce, to apply for legal status in the United States. She can independently obtain legal residency for herself and her children. The fear of deportation and loss of children who have been born in the United States is a primary reason for scores of undocumented women to remain in their abusive marriages (see the resource list at the end of this chapter).

MARIA (CONTINUED)

The nurse asked where my children were, and I told her they were at home with the neighbor. She asked if I had any friends or family who could support me. She then asked if I wanted to speak to an "advocate." She explained it was someone who could help me take the steps for safety. My journey to safety began that night. Although I went home that night, and suffered many more beatings, that night marked the beginning for me. The nurse gave me a piece of paper with a 1-800 number. I was too afraid to take the whole brochure because my husband always searched my purse. A week later, I called the number. And many weeks after that, I found the courage to go and meet my advocate. She was so patient, and she understood my terror. Little by little, I began to prepare my way out. The advocate introduced me to many other people who were instrumental in obtaining my freedom from violence.

CLINICAL IMPLICATIONS

It is critically important to address the abused woman's concerns about her children. Often, children are the reason an abused woman stays in the violent relationship (Hoff, 1990) and also the reason she leaves (Acevedo, 2000; Davis & Srinivasan, 1995; Kirkwood, 1993). For many mothers, be it women of color or women from the dominant culture, children are central to their lives. Identity is rooted in the role of motherhood. In the case of abused women, ignoring the centrality of children will doom any effort to address their needs. It is imperative that the medical and mental health care providers be ever vigilant regarding the needs of the children and how these intersect with the choices made by the woman herself (Koverola & Morahan, 2001).

PROVIDING INFORMATION IN A SAFE FORMAT IS CRITICAL

Although it is important to provide informational packages about domestic violence in multiple languages, a nondescript phone number is often the only piece of documentation a victim can safely take with her during the initial stages of help seeking. Domestic violence brochures and posters are now available in many languages. Information on additional resources is included at the end of this chapter.

MARIA (CONTINUED)

My advocate introduced me to the psychologist. Without her encouragement, I would never have had the courage to see a psychologist. In my country, psychologists are only for "crazy people." I had pain, but I knew I was not crazy. My advocate also introduced me to other women who were living in violence. I was so nervous at first, but finally I found the courage to attend the first session. The support group became my lifeline. These women knew my story even before I told it, because they had lived it. Angelina was the one who really convinced me to leave my husband. She had stayed too long in her relationship, and the state took her children from her. They said she had "failed to protect them from his abuse." She warned me, "someone will report you and then the workers will come to your house. Leave him, before he hurts them too." Angelina's pain convinced me to leave. In my culture, divorce is not permitted. I felt guilty before God, but I knew that my friend Angelina was right. I knew that I would cease to live if anyone took my children. In fact, that was partly why I had stayed. My husband had threatened that I would lose them if I left him.

CLINICAL IMPLICATIONS

Maria's case illustrates how important it was for the advocate and the psychologist to work with her on the intersection of domestic violence and the traditional cultural beliefs that Maria held about commitment to marriage before God. To be able to effectively intervene, the therapist must have an understanding of and respect for the cultural beliefs of the client (Lavizzo-Mourey & Mackenzie, 1996) and engage in a multifaceted, broad-based approach (Pinn & Chunko, 1997; Shea et al., 1997).

It is critical for the professional to realize the pivotal role of other survivors from similar circumstances, who speak the same language and share the same cultural traditions. The importance of facilitating engagement with a culturally appropriate support group cannot be overemphasized (Kanuha, 1994).

The example of Maria illustrates that the psychological distress and symptomatology manifested by women of color is often very similar to that documented in the dominant culture. It may, however, be described in different ways. For example, the distress may be described in a religious or cultural framework. Once the client is engaged in the process of intervention, many of the traditional approaches to intervening with disorders such as posttraumatic stress disorder can be implemented. Maria's story, however, illustrates that seeking the services of a psychologist holds tremendous negative stigma for many women of color. The critical linkage to the psychologist is typically made by means of a multidisciplinary team working in concert. Throughout this book, chapter authors have highlighted the imperative that, to adequately meet the needs of victims of family violence, psychologists must work as part of a team. This is especially true when providing services to women of color (Kanuha, 1994; Koverola & Morahan, 2001; Pinn & Chunko, 1997; Shea et al., 1997).

MARIA (CONTINUED)

Eighteen months after meeting the nurse, I was finally ready to meet the attorney who could help with the legal paperwork to apply for my own green card. Step by step, I was able to move forward. With my safety plan in place, I decided to go to the shelter with my children. There began another phase of my healing. It was a shelter where there were many other people who spoke Spanish. They even had our traditional foods. For the first time since leaving my parents, I felt safe. From the shelter, I finally found the courage to write the truth to my parents.

My road to healing began four years ago, and it has been a long, slow, and steady one. I have obtained a divorce, my immigration papers, a real job, and have rented my own apartment. I now volunteer at the shelter, and speak words of encouragement to my sisters who are trying to break free.

CLINICAL IMPLICATIONS

A critical component to working with women of color is to be able to provide contacts to practical legal resources needed to break out of their life of violence. It is important for practitioners to forge relationships with attorneys who can provide free or low-cost services to their clients as well as attorneys who speak the native languages of their clients. The legal needs of a woman leaving a violent relationship are often complex. Legal issues include obtaining restraining orders, filing for separation or divorce, custody issues, and financial issues. If there is child abuse, the mother may also be dealing with dependency court issues, which raises another whole host of legal concerns. The legal issues are even more complex when she resides in the United States illegally. It is important for practitioners to have an appreciation of the myriad legal issues faced by their clients and be able to direct them to appropriate resources.

The role of shelters is pivotal for many women leaving violent families. Increasingly, many shelters are developing specialized services for women of color, recognizing the importance of providing culturally appropriate shelter services (Kanuha, 1994). Professionals should be aware of these resources within their community. In smaller communities, the domestic violence shelter may not have the resources or numbers to develop specialized cultural services. In these situations, it is often possible to facilitate linkages between shelters and communities of faith or other cultural groups that collectively may provide additional support and resources to clients. In times of tremendous stress, as when a woman makes the choice to leave a violent relationship, she will benefit from being surrounded with familiar customs, rituals, foods, and so forth (Kanuha, 1994; West, 1998). Meeting the needs of women of color requires creativity and passion on the part of all who participate in the endeavor.

TANYA

I am a 30-year-old African American woman who was raised in the projects. I don't remember a time when my life did not include violence. I was first taken from my mother when I was 5 by a White lady. She kept saying "this was best." During the next 10 years, I lived in 15 foster homes. I was 12 the first time I was raped. It was one of my foster fathers. No one believed me, because of course by then I had a reputation as a liar. I never did get to see my own momma ever again, or my brothers and sisters. At night I'd cry for them, quietly so I wouldn't get whooped or teased. The first boy who loved me, he was in the last home—Jones. Jones has been in and out of my life ever since. We have four children together. I've always loved Jones and believe that he loved me. But he also beat me. They were bad beatings. He would just lose it and pulverize me. But letting go of Jones has been hard. How could I turn him in to the authorities? He's been charged with offenses he never did. He never had a decent attorney defend him. I'm the only one that was ever in his corner. No one has ever believed in Jones. Just me. I knew that when I finally turned my back on him, there would be no one there for Jones. Just the system that has been trying to take him down for the past decade. I felt such guilt. How could I turn on my own? It was easy to minimize and deny the abuse. In the end, I did have to turn my back on Jones, to save my own soul and the lives of my children.

CLINICAL IMPLICATIONS

Tanya's story reminds one of the complexities of dealing with discrimination and racism. For women from African American communities, abuse experiences need to be placed in the context of their experiences with racism and sexism. Abused African American women bear the dual burden of abuse and the common struggle, along with their partners, against racism. As a consequence, they are often under great pressure from their communities to overlook abusive acts of their partners, who presumably are displacing workplace frustration against discrimination (Oliver, 2000).

Thompson et al. (2000) found that African American women who reported partner violence experienced higher psychological distress and perceived themselves as having low levels of "emotional, informational, and tangible social support" (p. 137). Asbury (1987) discussed at length the complexity of seeking help as an African American. She noted that although studies have documented that women of all ethnic backgrounds are reluctant to reveal their abuse out of concern for their abusers, this may be an even greater concern for African American women. It is well established that African American men are in a more vulnerable position than other men relative to the dominant culture (Cazenave, 1981; Hare, 1979). African American women, being acutely aware of this oppression, may be very reluctant to expose them further. Asbury further noted that African American women may also be reluctant to bring attention to their situation if they have internalized very negative, but common, stereotypes about African American women. White (1980) noted that although many African American women have had to exhibit strength and independence for their own survival, this image may be problematic for those who find themselves in violent relationships.

MIN

I am a 35-year-old Chinese American mother of two. I am a physician. For 10 years, my husband physically and sexually assaulted me on a daily basis. My husband was a highly regarded physician in our community and ran for political office. For years, I lived in fear and silence, certain that no one would believe my story. My mother saw my bruises, but even she turned a deaf ear. She had lived the same life and believed it was our destiny. Honor, it was all about honor. I must not bring shame to the family. In those days, I often contemplated suicide. But I could not bring myself to it only because of my children.

Quite fortuitously, I heard about a psychologist who specialized in treating health professionals. I had developed panic attacks and made an appointment to see her to deal with this issue. Out tumbled my story. I paid cash for my sessions. I wanted no record of anything. My need for privacy was immense. My journey has been a slow one. Through psychotherapy, I learned about the dynamics of violence. I learned how it impacted me and the children. I explored how my cultural values and beliefs kept me hostage. Slowly, ever so slowly, I began to courageously heal. With the support of my therapist and my new circle of friends, I began to value my worth and dignity as a human being. It was very difficult because there were few within my cultural community that I could share my experience with because of how tightly knit the Chinese community actually is. Also, the fact that both my husband and I were physicians placed me in a situation of intense isolation because of the stature afforded physicians. Most of my support came from a group of other women professionals who had been in domestic violence relationships. As I began to become psychologically whole, my husband's capacity to control me diminished. He began to realize that he could no longer control me, and he moved on to other women, freeing me to be alone with my children. We are now legally separated.

CLINICAL IMPLICATIONS

It is important to be aware of the plight of educated women of color, who seemingly would have many resources but often are even more entrapped than their uneducated sisters living in poverty (Comas-Diaz & Greene, 1994). Min's story highlights again the cultural barriers faced by many women of color. Although Min had her own family here in the United

States, because of cultural pressures she was completely isolated from them. The pressure to suffer honorably, to not bring shame, kept her isolated and in pain. Psychotherapy allowed her to regain her sense of self and yet maintain some connection within her cultural community. Min was able to obtain support within her professional community.

Min's story highlights the cultural issue of maintaining honor that is so prominent within Asian cultures (Ho, 1990). This cultural barrier prevents many Asian women from seeking assistance for domestic violence. Within the American Indian culture, a related barrier is that of an "endurance of misfortune." LaFromboise, Berman, and Sohi (1994) wrote about how American Indians embrace this sense of ongoing misfortune—that one cannot fight it, nor should one fight it. This belief system makes it very difficult for an American Indian woman to seek assistance in ending the violence in her family. Comas-Diaz (1995) wrote about the "cultural fatalism"—a belief that certain negative life events happen regardless of efforts to prevent them—experienced by many Puerto Ricans. All of these are examples of how cultural barriers can impede help seeking by women of color.

BEWARE OF THE HOMOGENEITY MYTH

A chapter highlighting practice guidelines for ethnic minority clients would be remiss without a note on the *homogeneity myth* It is important for practitioners to understand the tremendous heterogeneity within minority groups. A common error made, particularly by individuals new to cross-cultural practice, is to assume homogeneity. Kaufman Kantor, Jasinski, and Aldarondo (1994) and Koverola (1996) have provided strong evidence confirming the heterogeneity within ethnic groups. Some have argued that there is as much within-group variance as between-group variance.

The issue is further complicated by the process of *acculturation*, that is, the extent to which an immigrant group takes on the norms and behavior patterns of the host society (Gordon, 1964). Kaufman Kantor et al. (1994) specifically investigated issues of acculturation among Hispanic families who had a history of marital violence. Their findings did not support a cultural mechanism for the transmission of abuse against women but rather provided evidence for cultural strengths as possible buffers against abuse.

The majority of the Vietnamese immigrant women in Bui and Morash's (1999) qualitative study reported a greater likelihood of embracing both American and Vietnamese cultures, and less belief in traditional roles, compared with the reports of their husbands' viewpoints. Conflicts arising out of the wives' changing norms and values in the new environment were significantly related to physical and emotional abuse of immigrant Vietnamese women (Bui & Morash, 1999). However, although the majority of the respondents in the study recognized that family violence was not a private matter in the United States, unlike in Vietnam, most abused women did not seek recourse from the criminal justice system because they feared arrest and racial discrimination against their husbands. Similarly, Acevedo's (2000) study underscored the importance of cultural factors in immigrant Mexican women's tolerance for abuse and the role of concrete help in recognition of abuse in their decisions to leave abusive relationships.

In their study of intimate violence among women of Mexican origin, Mattson and Rodriguez (1999) found that higher acculturation and acculturation stress, in the presence of other stressors, lack of support, and ability to cope, were significantly related to violence against women. In their traditional settings, families experience close bonds with family members, stability, and high social support. However, migration results in social isolation, disruption of traditional familial roles and role performance, and increased stress resulting from vastly different experiences in the new environment. Moreover, cultural prescriptions of indirect communication styles and stigma about abuse disclosure may prevent abused women from seeking help from sources other than familiar family networks (Bui & Morash, 1999; Firestone et al., 1999).

EVIDENCE-BASED PRACTICE?

In this chapter we have provided numerous practice recommendations for working with women of color who are victims of domestic violence. How many of these recommendations are evidence based? In a word: few. Despite 20 years of research on domestic violence, there is actually very little research that has been conducted specifically with ethnic minorities (West, 1998).

The research on domestic violence and ethnic minorities to date is primarily epidemiological in nature, confirming that it does indeed occur in all ethnic minority groups. However, there are very limited data on the differential health effects in ethnic minority victims of domestic violence. As is evident from the preceding discussion, there is some degree of consensus about "best practices" among practitioners who provide services to victims of violence who are women of color. Nevertheless, the gaps in research are self-evident. The National Institutes of Health has expanded guidelines to mandate the inclusion in its clinical trials of women from all ethnic and racial backgrounds. This, together with an increased recognition of the importance of socioeconomic and psychosocial factors in health and disease, has strengthened efforts to improve understanding of domestic violence in diverse communities (Pinn & Chunko, 1997). These research efforts, however, are only now being launched, and the findings are not yet available.

FINAL COMMENT

Maria, Tanya, and Min represent the collective voices of thousands of women of color who are survivors of domestic violence. Although there are similarities among them, each story is unique; each woman is an individual. We encourage medical and mental health practitioners not only to listen attentively to women of color who come to them but also to remember the ones who do not come but rather need professionals to reach out to them. Women of color who are victims of domestic violence face seemingly insurmountable barriers. Be a person who reaches out beyond those barriers.

ADDITIONAL RESOURCES

National Coalition Against Domestic Violence Hotline: 1-800-799-7233

Family Violence Prevention Fund: http://www.fvpf.org

Family Research Laboratory at the University of New Hampshire: http://www.unh.edu/frl

Minnesota Center Against Violence and Abuse: http://www.mincava.umn.edu

National Criminal Justice Reference Service: http://www.ncjrs.org

Asian and Pacific Islander American Health forum; has links to articles regarding domestic violence against these minority women: http://www.apiahf.org

South Asian Women's Network: http://www.sawnet.org

Information on the Violence Against Women Act, and application for amnesty, is available on the following Web sites: http://www.ins.usdoj.gov/graphics/howdoi/battered.htm and http://www.ojp.usdoj.gov/vawo/laws/vawa/vawa.htm

REFERENCES

Acevedo, M. J. (2000). Battered immigrant Mexican women's perspectives regarding abuse and help-seeking. *Journal of Multicultural Social Work, 8,* 243–282.

Almeida, R. V., & Dolan-Delvecchio, K. (1999). Addressing culture in batterers intervention: The Asian Indian community as an illustrative example. *Violence Against Women, 5,* 654–683.

Almeida, R. V., & Durkin, T. (1999). The cultural context model: Therapy for couples with domestic violence. *Journal of Marital and Family Therapy, 25,* 313–324.

Asbury, J. E. (1987). African-American women in violent relationships: An exploration of cultural differences. In R. L. Hampton (Ed.), *Violence in the Black family: Correlates and consequences* (pp. 89–105). Lexington, MA: Lexington Books.

Baker, N. (1999). Family killing fields: Honor rationales in the murder of women. *Violence Against Women, 5,* 164–184.

Barnes, S. Y. (1999). Theories of spouse abuse: Relevance to African Americans. *Issues in Mental Health Nursing, 20*, 357–371.

Bohn, D. K., & Holz, K. A. (1996). Sequelae of abuse: Health effects of childhood sexual abuse, domestic battering, and rape. *Journal of Nurse-Midwifery, 41*, 442–456.

Bui, H. N., & Morash, M. (1999). Domestic violence in the Vietnamese immigrant community: An exploratory study. *Violence Against Women, 5*, 769–795.

Campbell, J. C., Pliska, M. J., Taylor, W., & Sheridan, D. (1994). Battered women's experiences in the emergency department. *Journal of Emergency Nursing, 20*, 280–288.

Cazenave, N. A. (1981). Black men in America: The quest for manhood. In H. P. McAdoo (Ed.), *Black families* (pp. 176–185). Beverly Hills, CA: Sage.

Comas-Diaz, L. (1995). Puerto Ricans and sexual child abuse. In L. A. Fontes (Ed.), *Sexual abuse in nine North American cultures: Treatment and prevention* (pp. 31–66). Thousand Oaks, CA: Sage.

Comas-Diaz, L., & Greene, B. (1994). *Women of color: Integrating ethnic and gender identities in psychotherapy.* New York: Guilford Press.

Davis, L. V., & Srinivasan, M. (1995). Listening to the voices of battered women: What helps them escape violence. *Affilia, 10*, 49–69.

Fanslow, J. L., Norton, R. N., & Spinola, C. G. (1998). Indicators of assault-related injuries among women presenting to the emergency department. *Annals of Emergency Medicine, 32*, 341–348.

Feldhaus, K. M., Koziol-McLain, J., Amsbury, H. L., Norton, I. M., Lowenstein, S. R., & Abbott, J. T. (1997). Accuracy of three brief screening questions for detecting partner violence in the emergency department. *Journal of the American Medical Association, 277*, 1357–1361.

Firestone, J. M., Lambert, L. C., & Vega, W. A. (1999). Intimate violence among women of Mexican origin: Correlates of abuse. *Journal of Gender, Culture, and Health, 4*, 119–134.

Gordon M. (1964). *Assimilation in American life: The role of race, religion and national origins.* New York: Oxford University Press.

Hall, D., & Lynch, M. A. (1998). Violence begins at home. *British Medical Journal, 316*, 1551–1560.

Hare, N. (1979). The relative psycho-socio-economic suppression of the Black male. In W. D. Smith et al. (Ed.), *Reflections on Black psychology* (pp. 359–381). Washington, DC: University Press of America.

Ho, C. K. (1990). An analysis of domestic violence in Asian American communities: A multicultural approach to counseling. In L. S. Brown & M. Root (Eds.), *Diversity and complexity in feminist therapy* (pp. 129–150). New York: Harrington Park.

Hoff, L. A. (1990). *Battered women as survivors.* London: Routledge.

Kanuha, V. (1994). Women of color in battering relationships. In L. Comas-Diaz & B. Greene (Eds.), *Women of color: Integrating ethnic and gender identities in psychotherapy* (pp. 428–454). New York: Guilford Press.

Kaufman Kantor, G., Jasinski, J. L., & Aldarondo, E. (1994). Sociocultural status and incidence of marital violence in Hispanic families. *Violence and Victims, 9,* 207–222.

Kirkwood, C. (1993). *Leaving abusive partners.* London: Sage.

Koverola, C. (1996). Counseling Aboriginal people of North America. *Journal of Psychology and Christianity, 11,* 345–357.

Koverola, C., & Morahan, M. (2001). Children exposed to domestic violence. In C. Green-Hernandez, J. K. Singleton, & D. Z. Aronzon (Eds.), *Primary care pediatrics* (pp. 275–281). Philadelphia: Lippincott.

LaFromboise, T. D., Berman, J. S., & Sohi, B. K. (1994). American Indian women: Identities in psychotherapy. In L. Comas-Diaz & B. Greene (Eds.), *Women of color: Integrating ethnic and gender identities in psychotherapy* (pp. 30–71). New York: Guilford Press.

Lavizzo-Mourey, R., & Mackenzie, E. R. (1996). Cultural competence: Essential measurements of quality for managed care organizations. *Annals of Internal Medicine, 124,* 919–921.

Lawson, E. J., Rodgers-Rose, L. F., & Rajaram, S. (1999). The psychosocial context of Black women's health. *Health Care for Women International, 20,* 279–289.

Mattson, S., & Rodriguez, E. (1999). Battering in pregnant Latinas. *Issues in Mental Health Nursing, 20,* 405–422.

McGee, M. P. (1997). Cultural values and domestic violence. *Journal of Family Social Work, 2,* 129–140.

Oliver, W. (2000). Preventing domestic violence in the African American community. *Violence Against Women, 6,* 533–549.

Pinn, V. W., & Chunko, M. T. (1997). The diverse faces of violence: Minority women and domestic abuse. *Academic Medicine, 72,* S65–S71.

Segal, U. A. (2000). A pilot exploration of family violence among non-clinical Vietnamese. *Journal of Interpersonal Violence, 15,* 523–533.

Shea, C. A., Mahoney, M., & Lacey, J. M. (1997). Breaking through the barriers to domestic violence intervention. *American Journal of Nursing, 97*(6), 26–34.

Thompson, M. P., Kaslow, N. J., Kingree, J. B., Rashid, A., Puett, R., Jacobs, D., & Matthews, A. (2000). Partner violence, social support, and distress among inner-city African American women. *American Journal of Community Psychology, 28,* 127–143.

U.S. Department of Health and Human Services, National Institutes of Health. (1994, March 28). NIH Guidelines on the Inclusion of Women and Minorities as Subjects in Clinical Research; Notice, 59 Fed Reg. 14,508–15,413.

U.S. Department of Health and Human Services, Public Health Office, Office of the Surgeon General. (2001). *Mental health: Culture, race and ethnicity—A supplement to mental health: A report of the Surgeon General. Executive summary.* Rockville, MD: Author.

West, C. (1998). Lifting the "political gag order": Breaking the silence around partner violence in ethnic minority families. In J. Jasinski & L. Williams (Eds.), *Partner violence: A comprehensive review of 20 years of research* (pp. 184–209). Thousand Oaks, CA: Sage.

White, J. L. (1980). Toward a black psychology. In R. L. Jones (Ed.), *Black Psychology* (pp. 5–12). New York: HarperCollins.

Zink, T. (2000). Should children be in the room when the mother is screened for partner violence? *Journal of Family Practice, 49,* 130–136.

4

WHY HEALTH CARE PROFESSIONALS ARE RELUCTANT TO INTERVENE IN CASES OF ONGOING DOMESTIC ABUSE

L. KEVIN HAMBERGER AND DARSHANA PATEL

Domestic violence often presents in health care settings, yet health care professionals sometimes miss obvious signs or fail to ask about abuse. Lack of training, the belief that domestic abuse is none of their business, and lack of system support are all reasons why domestic violence is often not identified. Clinicians may also have personal reasons for their lack of intervention, including lack of comfort with the topic or negative beliefs about women who are domestically abused. This chapter describes these barriers and offers practical steps clinicians can take to overcome them.

Mrs. WT, a 32-year-old woman, presents to Dr. JK's office five months after her preterm delivery for a postpartum checkup with complaints of not feeling well and wanting a prescription to increase her energy. She is also requesting sleeping medicine and a referral for tubal ligation. Mrs. WT describes to Dr. JK that lately she has been feeling very tired and not able to get enough sleep with three kids and her husband's odd work schedule. She says she has to pay lots of attention to her sick premature son, Joey.

Mrs. WT apologizes for missing a few appointments since Joey's birth. She is very concerned about her ability to give enough care to all her kids because sometimes she gets impatient with her older daughters, aged 7 and 3 years.

Mrs. WT had worked as a secretary in a local law firm, but because of the sudden and early delivery of Joey at 29 weeks of pregnancy, and his poor health, Mrs. WT had to quit. Mrs. WT accepts help from her neighbors and church friends. However, 7-year-old Lisa often misses school so she can help with domestic chores and child care.

Mrs. WT's husband, Mr. XT, is a truck driver and is frequently gone for days. Mrs. WT states that her husband's work is very stressful and that she tries to make his life easier when he is home. She says that many a time, no matter how hard she tries, it is not enough.

Dr. JK has known Mrs. WT since the birth of her second daughter, Mary, three years ago. He has asked her a screening question for domestic violence in the past and even during the recent pregnancy. Mrs. WT has a very good rapport with Dr. JK. Dr. JK is also a family physician for Mr. XT and the three children. Mr. XT is a very caring and charming husband and father. During today's visit, Mrs. WT looks anxious, avoids eye contact while talking, and is not well groomed.

> Dr. JK: Is everything OK at home?
> Mrs. WT: [avoids eye contact] Yes.
> Dr. JK: How is your relationship with your husband?
> Mrs. WT: Fine.
> Dr. JK: Is there anything that I can help you with?
> Mrs. WT: No. I just need a vitamin and a sleeping pill.

Even though Dr. JK felt that there was some tension in Mrs. WT's relationship with her husband, he could not ask her specific questions about it, so he did not get a specific answer. Dr. JK recalled what he learned during his training on domestic violence screening and intervention and how to overcome the barriers encountered. He tried another approach:

> Due to your husband's work schedule, and your new adjustments with a premature baby, let's talk about the stresses you are experiencing in your relationship. In my experience, a new premature baby, financial difficulty, and a partner's new work schedule many a time cause relationship strain. Are you experiencing any emotional or verbal strain in your relationship? Is your husband calling you names or putting you down? In the last year, has he physically or sexually hurt you? Did he make you feel afraid for your or your children's safety in the last year?

Mrs. WT attended to what Dr. JK asked and replied, "Lately, my husband is becoming more demanding and impatient with me. I try so hard, but it doesn't seem to satisfy him." She cried as she said he accuses her of sleeping around when he is gone: "He gets so suspicious when he comes back from his long-distance driving assignment. He checks the whole apartment for any signs of anyone being there while he was out." Lately, he disconnected the long-distance carrier so that she cannot even call her sister, who lives in a nearby state.

> He calls me in the middle of the night just to make sure that I am home and not with anyone else! He even questions my older daughter about anyone else being there. I have repeatedly told him that I love him, and I cannot think about going out with anyone else. But he seems not to understand it.

She continues, "He then gives me some made-up examples how other truck drivers lost their partners, and says I should feel lucky that he is not going out with someone else while he is away."

Dr. JK validated her experience, saying, "You don't deserve to be treated this way. You are not alone. I give you credit for sharing this very delicate issue. We have help available."

Mrs. WT felt relieved that she was not judged but was empathetically heard and was directed to a nearby women's resource center for further help. Dr. JK assured Mrs. WT that all the information given to him is confidential and that under no circumstances would he disclose it to her husband. Dr. JK felt relieved that his training in domestic violence screening helped him to overcome the barrier he personally felt in asking direct screening questions and confidently providing support and referral in a nonjudgmental manner.

SCREENING FOR DOMESTIC VIOLENCE IN HEALTH CARE SETTINGS

In recent years, several medical and mental health professionals called for the screening of all female patients for domestic violence and, if they are thus identified, for helping them (Ambuel, Hamberger, & Lahti, 1997; McLeer, Anwar, Herman, & Maquiling, 1989; Stark & Flitcraft, 1996). Because women frequently seek services in primary care, obstetrical, and emergency settings, these sites seem ideal for domestic violence screening (Thompson, et al., 2000). To best reach women in such settings, researchers and scholars advocate for universal domestic violence screening (Ambuel et al., 1997; Stark & Flitcraft, 1996). Although, as we show later in this chapter, universal screening is controversial for a number of reasons, it is preferred to case finding (i.e., waiting for signs or symptoms before asking about domestic violence), because there is no known medical or psychosocial syndrome of battering that is specific and sensitive such that providers can wait for the requisite syndrome to implement domestic violence screening.

Domestic violence screening can take many forms: patient self-report, health information forms, or questions about partner violence in the clinical interview during history taking. Professionals can also screen while asking about psychosocial aspects of illness or when asking prevention-related questions. Screening conducted by means of an interview provides a higher positive yield than do written, self-report approaches (Gazmararian et al., 1996). Hence, advocates of universal screening favor interview-style screening approaches, despite potential implementation problems.

As health care providers, psychologists can join their medical colleagues in efforts to screen female patients for partner violence. First, psychologists can conduct screening in their own practices. Second, they can participate in development of curricula to train other health care providers to screen and help partner violence victims. Third, they can help evaluate screening and intervention efforts. Finally, psychologists can use their evaluation and assessment skills to identify and overcome the many barriers health care providers face in screening and helping partner violence victims.

BARRIERS TO SCREENING, IDENTIFICATION, AND HELPING DOMESTIC VIOLENCE VICTIMS

Health care providers, psychologists in health care settings, and patients face many barriers to screening, identifying, and helping patients who are trapped in violent and abusive intimate relationships. Barriers can be unique to the health care provider, the patient, and the overall health care system.

Health Care Provider Barriers

Lack of Knowledge

Perhaps the most typically identified barrier for health care providers is lack of education. Sugg & Inui (1992) reported that among their sample of primary care physicians, 61% reported not having had previous training in domestic violence. Hamberger et al. (in press) found that nearly 50% of nursing staff, with an average career duration of 14 years, working at a community-based medical system did not have prior training in domestic violence. Although in recent years more medical schools and residency programs have developed and included in their core curricula family violence education (Hendricks-Matthews, 1991), such training is variable in terms of quantity and quality. For example, Short, Cotton, and Hodgson (1997) described a comprehensive and carefully tested domestic violence module for medical students. In contrast, Phelan, Melzer-Lange, Hamberger, and Ambuel (2000) and Melzer-Lange, Phelan, Hamberger, and Ambuel (2000) described a medical school curriculum survey that suggested wide but variable coverage of child abuse, partner abuse, and elder abuse. In the area of mental health training, the breadth and depth of curricular coverage of domestic violence are not known; hence, even though professional schools and specialty disciplines have increased training in domestic violence, significant gaps continue to exist, leaving health care providers unprepared to screen, identify, and help victims of partner violence.

The most basic educational and knowledge deficit includes a lack of overall knowledge about domestic violence, such as a working definition of domestic violence, its dynamics, and the prevalence of victims and survivors within a typical practice specialty. For such providers, domestic violence is "not on the radar screen," and they are unlikely to ask patients about it at all. Such providers may assume that their communities and patients do not have such problems.

A related skill deficit is how to screen for domestic violence in clinical practice. Providers may possess some knowledge about domestic violence but lack the understanding of and skill in asking about it in such a way as to put patients at ease and facilitate valid responses (Gerbert et al., 1996).

A third knowledge and skill deficit is in performing the complex set of responses to patients who either report living in an abusive relationship or show many positive signs of doing so but deny it. Providers frequently object to screening on the basis that they will not know what to say or do if a patient responds positively to screening. They further reason that if they do not know how to respond in a helpful and therapeutic way to a positive report, they are ethically bound to not open up the subject with their patients.

Fear of Offending Patients

Health care providers frequently fear that their patients will be offended when asked about domestic abuse. However, Hamberger, Ambuel, Marbella, and Donze (1998) found that battered women wanted their physicians to ask about domestic violence. Furthermore, among primary-care patients not selected because of a background in domestic violence, 78% favored routine domestic violence inquiry. When such questions are couched within other questions related to prevention and safety, and presented in a matter-of-fact manner, there is little reason to believe that most patients will be offended.

Perceived Time Pressures

Health care providers also frequently cite time pressure as a major barrier to asking about partner violence. In focus groups with health care providers to identify barriers to screening, Minsky, Pape, and Hamberger (2000) reported that many participants described feeling overworked and overwhelmed with their current staffing responsibilities and patterns. They viewed domestic violence screening and intervention as a major impediment to performing their other duties in a positive and professional manner. Indirect time pressure concerns included concerns about tying up rooms needed to maintain patient flow as other staff worked with patients who admitted to abuse. This reduced physician productivity and increased staff overtime, thus increasing costs.

Perceived Irrelevance of Domestic Violence to Health Care Practice

Despite evidence that domestic violence is a legitimate and important health care issue, many providers view it as outside their purview (Fletcher, 1994). Minsky et al. (2000) found that many respondents failed to understand or accept responsibility for screening, as summarized by the following rhetorical question: "How much responsibility do I own to save the world?"

A variation of this attitude is the notion that domestic violence screening is relevant, but not to one's particular medical specialty and setting. For example, Minsky et al. (2000) found that staff working in a labor and delivery unit strongly believed that domestic violence posed significant dangers to both mother and child; however, they also opined that domestic violence screening should have occurred during prenatal visits. They expressed concern that because their patients were primarily in active labor, screening was irrelevant to their immediate tasks of facilitating delivery. Similarly, emergency department staff acknowledged the potential damage to patients from domestic violence and the importance that medical staff identify and assist battered victims, if possible, but they expressed concern about the relevance of universal screening (Minsky et al., 2000). Instead, staff preferred to screen for domestic violence only in situations in which patients presented clinical evidence of being in a violent relationship, such as a suspicious injury pattern or depressed mood.

Fear of Loss of Control of the Provider–Patient Relationship

Many primary-care physicians fear that once domestic violence is identified, a chain of events will be set off that will wrest control of the entire encounter from the physician (Sugg & Inui, 1992). Included in this Pandora's box are strong patient emotional responses, time spent in crisis management, loss of control over the rest of the schedule, fear of litigation, fear of reprisal by the abusive spouse, and inability to control the outcome for the patient. This fear of loss of control is important to health care providers, who are accustomed to following protocols and treatment guidelines. They are trained to assess, diagnose, and prescribe treatment. Domestic violence does not lend itself neatly to such a model (Warshaw, 1989). Working with domestic violence victims requires a collaboration that validates the victims' experiences and trusts that they make decisions about safety and survival that are rational and strategic, even if, to an outsider, the decisions may appear otherwise. If control of the intervention process is the primary value, such collaboration cannot occur, and thus appropriate screening or intervention behaviors will not take place.

Provider Attitudes and Accountability

Health care providers sometimes exhibit attitudes and behaviors that directly inhibit screening, identification, and help of abuse victims. Moore, Zaccaro, and Parsons (1998) identified victim blaming as one such attitude. Another attitude is that some physical violence is to be expected in families. Still others include concern about patient truthfulness in reporting abuse and not viewing abuse as a medical problem or as the provider's business. Rodriguez, Bauer, McLoughlin, and Grumbach (1999) identified physician victim-blaming attitudes including blaming patients for failure to disclose abuse and failure to follow up with referrals and recommendations. Hamberger et al. (1998) reported on a small but notable percentage of physicians who blamed the victim through jokes and hostile expressions. Other research has shown that battered women in emergency departments are treated differently, depending on whether they appeared to be intoxicated, psychiatrically ill, or unconventional (Kurz, 1987; Larkin, Hyman, Mathias, D'Amico, and MacLeod, 1999).

Larkin, Rolniak, Hyman, MacLeod, and Savage (2000) showed that after screening was formalized as part of a job description and screening compliance was included in quarterly performance reviews, screening rates increased significantly. Pape, Minsky, and Hamberger (2000) found that feedback to clinical departments about screening rates relative to set goals resulted in consistent, higher screening rates.

Provider Discomfort

For a number of health care providers, the issue of domestic violence creates sufficient discomfort that they avoid dealing with it professionally as much as possible (Sugg & Inui, 1992). Ambuel et al. (1997) noted that both providers who have firsthand experience with family violence and those who do not may find the issue overwhelming. For many of these individuals, survivor stories, whether provided in person or in videotaped accounts during training, are shocking and emotionally overwhelming. Ambuel, Butler, Hamberger, Lawrence, and Guse (2003) also identified a certain percentage who could not feel comfortable asking or helping partner violence victims in medical practice; they were too distressed and depressed about their own experiences to feel confident or motivated to help others in similar situations. Such feelings obviously constitute a significant barrier.

After conducting training workshops, we have had such "uninitiated" learners relate strong emotional reactions that included nightmares and feelings of depression and anxiety. Without some opportunity for debriefing and processing intense feelings, such health care professionals may avoid screening and intervention activities.

Patient Barriers

Patients who struggle with intimate partner violence rarely volunteer or discuss such information with their health care providers (Plichta, Duncan, & Plichta, 1996). Although, as we discussed above, health care providers themselves create many barriers to disclosure, patients also create barriers to their own identification. It may seem that patients struggling with domestic violence should want to tell their health care providers about their plight; however, one must consider that battered victims create barriers to their identification as a survival mechanism designed to protect them, as well as their children, and even their abusive partners, from harm.

Lack of Trust

Although female victims of partner violence make significantly more visits for health care services (Stark et al., 1981), they are not likely to disclose the abuse to health care providers. McNutt, Carlson, Gagen, and Winterbauer (1999) found that of a sample of battered women from both medical and urban domestic violence programs, only 19% reported having volunteered to their health care provider that they had been battered. In addition, 20% reported that they actually denied being abused when asked. Such nondisclosure and overt denial are frequently intentional, strategic decisions (Gerbert et al., 1996). In particular, health care providers who appear uninterested or uncaring in their overall approach to the patient are perceived as not trustworthy by abuse victims.

Fear of Retribution

An issue related to trust is fear. For example, some patients fear that disclosing abuse to a health care provider can lead to abuser retribution. In medical settings, this can occur when a health care provider asks about domestic violence when other family members, including the possible perpetrator, are present. It can also occur when a well-meaning health care provider receives the information in private but, without the patient's consent, confronts the abuser in an effort to be helpful (Hamberger et al., 1998). Hansen, Harway, and Cervantes (1991) found a strong tendency among marriage and family therapists to treat information about domestic violence as evidence of an underlying communication problem, with a preference to treat the couple rather than to work with the victim alone and in confidence. Domestic violence is shrouded in isolation and secrecy. Battered victims are typically threatened with violence should they disclose the abuse.

Fear of Loss of Control

Abuse victims also frequently fear that disclosure of abuse will result in pressure to leave the relationship and lead down an inevitable path toward dissolution of the relationship and loss of the partner (Rodriguez, Craig, Mooney, & Bauer, 1998). This, in turn, can lead to other negative, albeit unintended consequences. Ending a relationship and moving out can be one of the most dangerous times in the life of a battered victim, with a potential risk of severe injury and homicide. Other related fears include loss of financial support, particularly if the perpetrator is the primary wage earner (Brown, Lent, & Sas, 1993; Rodriguez et al., 1998). Even with continued financial support, maintenance of separate households results in a decreased standard of living for the victim and the perpetrator. Hence, unless the patient is given strong assurances that screening and possible disclosure will result in a collaborative plan for safety, and not prescriptions to leave the relationship, a victim is not likely to acknowledge abuse.

Many victims will also not disclose for fear of losing child custody (Rodriguez et al., 1998). This could happen in a number of ways. If the clinician determines that the children in the home are also at risk for abuse, he or she may decide to report the situation to a child protective services agency, triggering an investigation and possible removal of the children from the household. Abuse victims could also lose custody of their children through custody suits. Batterers punish their partners through such actions, and they frequently win. Such suits also assure that the victim will have to interact in various ways with the batterer long after the relationship is over. These fears are also part of the calculus victims use in determining whether they will answer affirmatively a screening question about abuse.

Sense of Futility

Domestic violence is a pattern of coercion and control that pervades every aspect of victims' lives. Over time, most victims have made many attempts to end the violence, including appeasement, fighting back, going to counseling for themselves and for the relationship, seeking spiritual support, calling police, and reaching out to family and friends. Each time, they may have met with failure. They discovered that appeasement led to other reasons to batter. Fighting back led to being beaten even harder or even arrest for "abuse." If they reached out to family or friends, they may have been repelled for going against advice or chastised for disloyalty to their partners. The batterer may have also threatened friends and family, intimidating them and rendering them unhelpful. Spiritual leaders may have encouraged the victim to pray harder and, above all, to keep the family together (Miles, 2000). Counseling may have resulted in diagnoses, medication, and labels. Efforts to live independently may have met with failure because of financial constraints and lack of job readiness. After so many failures, battered women, as patients in a medical setting, might not disclose abuse. A health care provider's friendly and concerned inquiry, though well intentioned, is viewed as lacking credibility because the victim–patient does not know how the provider can help (Brown et al., 1993).

The Nature of the Intimate Relationship

The context of partner violence is also an important factor when considering why battered women do not always readily disclose that they are living in an abusive relationship. Abuse victims frequently report that they love their partners. They want the violence to end, not the relationship. Some abuse victims may not disclose out of a sense of loyalty to their partners. Dutton and Painter (1993) discussed this in terms of traumatic bonding. As time passes after an assault, the victim perceives the perpetrator and the relationship in a more positive light. Focusing on the positive aspects may also relate to a tendency to deny and minimize the level of violence and abuse.

A Problem of Expectations: What Providers and Patients Expect of Each Other

Some barriers to screening, identification, and helping battered victims could be a function of the provider–patient interaction—a "dance of disclosure and identification" (Gerbert, Abercrombie, Caspers, Love, & Bronstone, 1999, p. 122). That is, battered women offer a range of disclosures—from overt disclosures, to subtle hints, to lies—about their abuse. Their hopes range from being identified to fear that identification will lead to more violence. However, providers who are successful in this area make inquiries ranging from direct questions to hinting and indirect inquiries that are made over time. As the patient–victim feels increasingly confident that his or her provider will maintain confidentiality and possesses the skill to help he or she becomes more likely to disclose abuse. Panagiota and Musialowski (1997) found that 68% of women with abuse histories would be willing to tell their doctors if the doctors first asked. However, only 12% reported that they had been asked about domestic violence, and, of those who did tell their doctors of the abuse, 20% of the physicians did nothing about it. Plichta et al. (1996) found that, compared with nonbattered women, battered women reported more dissatisfaction with their doctor and poorer communication. These findings suggest that spouse abuse creates a barrier to doctor–patient communication that leads to lower patient satisfaction.

System-Level Barriers

In their review, Waalen, Goodwin, Spitz, Petersen, and Saltzman (2000) found that education about domestic violence and screening–intervention alone is not related to increases in screening and detection rates. Other factors intrinsic to the organizational system may inhibit or prevent effective screening and intervention. For example, McLeer and colleagues (1989) reported that inclusion of a systematic protocol for identification of abuse in an emergency department increased detection rates from approximately 5% to 30%. However, the system discontinued the protocol, and subsequent detection rates reverted to near-baseline levels. Roberts, Lawrence, O'Toole, and Raphael (1997) and Minsky et al. (2000) found that a system-level barrier that neutralized the effectiveness of education was lack of a referral network, or an on-site patient advocate, to help abused patients.

Minsky et al. (2000) conducted a qualitative study with focus groups from a number of health system departments that serve women. The results revealed a number of systemic barriers that inhibited or precluded screening and intervention, even among health care providers who valued such tasks and services. A major systemic barrier identified by several departments was time pressures and high workloads, which we discussed earlier.

Many providers also suggested that although the organization was committed to train all staff about domestic violence, there was insufficient systemic support to create the infrastructure to support such work in the trenches. Specifically, staff identified insufficient physical space that offered privacy for screening and intervention, particularly in emergency settings. Another system barrier was lack of a process to give providers feedback on patient outcomes. Providers expressed concern and consternation that, without feedback about the adequacy of their interventions, they were reluctant to invest more time and effort in the activity, particularly in an atmosphere of competing demands.

Is the Total Environment Domestic Violence Competent?

There are little, if any, data on the type of total environment that communicates to abuse victims that a particular system or clinical setting is a safe place to disclose and receive help for domestic violence. As noted above, provider and clinic/system credibility will be developed and earned over time through numerous encounters among providers, allied staff, reception staff, and others whom the patient–victim encounters. Clinics that appear cold and uncaring about basic respect; privacy; and competent, compassionate health care may be viewed by victims as threatening to their safety should they disclose (Ambuel et al., 1997). In contrast, Hamberger et al. (1998) found that battered women's preferences for physician interactions with them were consistent with provision of compassionate, respectful, and humane health care. Such health care includes asking questions, performing thorough histories, conducting sensitive and gentle physical examinations, and completing documentation and follow-up.

Overcoming Barriers

Although many barriers to screening, identification, and intervention with abuse victims in medical settings exist, they can be overcome with appropriate interventions. Areas of intervention include education, use of protocols, administrative interventions, continuous quality improvement approaches, and patient-friendly clinic environments.

Role of Education

Although education alone has not been shown to significantly affect health care provider screening and intervention behavior, it does appear to be a necessary, if not sufficient, part of any initiative. In fact, some studies have shown a number of positive effects of education. For example, education has been shown to increase providers' self-efficacy in asking screening questions and providing appropriate help (Hamberger et al., in press; Harwell et al., 1998; Thompson et al., 2000). Such studies suggest that education can successfully address various health care provider barriers related to lack of education and skill and fear of offending or losing control of the provider–patient relationship. Education may also be necessary to help providers assess their roles and goals for screening and intervention. For example, after training, providers frequently express understanding of their limited role to screen, identify, and, within the scope of their professional practice, help victims (Hamberger et al., in press). Likewise, Gerbert et al. (1999) found that physicians who had developed expertise working with abused patients learned to redefine the concept of successful outcome from one of the patient taking immediate action to the asking of screening questions in a compassionate and respectful manner. Physicians who redefined success in this way transformed their sense of responsibility from making things happen to planting seeds and providing compassionate care— something they have been trained to do in all aspects of medical practice.

Some research has shown that health care providers do show increases in screening and interventional behavior after training (Harwell et al., 1998; Thompson et al., 2000). It is not currently known, however, what components of education are necessary to affect behavior change. Thompson et al. (2000), for example, used a comprehensive training program that consisted of two half-day training sessions, clinical educational rounds, booster educational sessions with selected leaders, and a bimonthly domestic violence newsletter. Providers were also given feedback on the results of their efforts and provided with systemic support in the form of posters and cue cards to facilitate screening and intervention. Harwell et al. (1998) reported a similarly comprehensive educational intervention program. Research is needed to identify key components of education that facilitate attitude and behavior change.

Impact of Protocols

Implementing written protocols or prompts has been found to significantly increase documented rates of screening and intervention with abuse victims (Waalen et al., 2000). McLeer et al. (1989) demonstrated that, after implementation of a screening protocol in an emergency department, identification rates increased about sixfold. Adding a screening prompt to the patient's chart resulted in significant increases in documented screening (Olson, Anctil, Fullerton, Brillman, Arbuckle, & Sklar, 1996). Patel, Hamberger, and Griffin (2001) found that documented rates of screening increased from 2% to 92% after inclusion of a screening question on the history form in a family practice setting. However, McGrath et al. (1997) cautioned that protocols alone, without education and appropriate institutional support to overcome barriers, do not result in increased screening and intervention.

Administrative Interventions

As described above, formally incorporating screening rates into providers' job descriptions and quarterly performance reviews significantly increased screening rates among nurses (Larkin et al., 2000). Pape et al. (2000) described a continuous quality improvement intervention that included setting screening rate goals; conducting regular, random chart audits; and providing feedback to clinical departments. Specialized in-service training and administrative troubleshooting were also implemented to address ongoing barriers and problems. The researchers found that the intervention resulted in significantly increased screening and referral rates. Kurz (1987) found that, compared with an emergency department that did not have a designated domestic violence advocate, the emergency department that did have one identified four times more victims.

Creating Victim-Friendly Clinical Environments

Although there is little specific research available on the topic, the literature suggests that victims and survivors are very observant of environmental cues that provide information about whether it is safe for them to disclose abuse (Gerbert et al., 1999). Bolin and Elliott (1996) found that when doctors trained in domestic violence wore buttons that read "It's OK to talk to me about family violence and abuse," significantly more patients initiated discussion about the topic than when buttons were not worn. This suggests that patients respond positively when health care systems communicate that its providers understand domestic violence and are trained and prepared to help in various, appropriate ways. Other ways clinic environments can communicate similar messages include stocking examination rooms and restrooms with posters and brochures about family violence, training all staff to be sensitive to partner violence, and training all direct-service staff to screen and provide emotional support to anyone who discloses domestic violence (Ambuel et al., 1997).

SUMMARY

Barriers to screen, identify, and help victims of partner violence are multifaceted and include health care providers, patients, the clinic environment, and, on a larger scale, the systems and communities in which health care is delivered. For providers, barriers to screen include lack of overall knowledge of domestic violence, personal discomfort and disbelief in domestic-violence dynamics, fear of legal consequences, fear of damaging the patient–provider relationship, lack of sufficient time, and perceived irrelevance of domestic violence in certain health care settings. For patients, barriers include lack of trust in the provider, fear of retribution and loss of financial support, loss of child custody, lack of social and family support, fear of losing the provider's respect, and fear of being mislabeled as mentally ill.

Domestic violence does not fit into the traditional model of disease identification, assessment, and treatment prescription. Providers must understand that domestic violence is a struggle of power in which the victim has lost control of many aspects of his or her life. A basic gift one can provide is to return decision-making control to the victim instead of prescribing specific actions, and this includes respecting the victim's autonomy and decisions. Although research has begun to identify the various barriers, less is known about interventions to address and overcome them. It does appear, however, that one-shot, short-term education programs alone are insufficient to affect large-scale change in domestic violence screening and intervention in health care settings. There is growing evidence that comprehensive intervention programs that incorporate education; clinical protocols and guidelines; and institutional support in the form of space and time, provider feedback, and accountability can result in increased identification of abuse victims. Unknown as yet are the minimal and optimal components of effective programs to facilitate these goals. In addition, although research is beginning to shed light on methods for increasing and supporting clinicians' efforts to intervene with abuse victims, a significant gap in the literature and knowledge base is the impact such interventions have on the lives of the intended beneficiaries.

REFERENCES

Ambuel, B., Butler, D., Hamberger, L. K., Lawrence, S., & Guse, C. (2003). Female and male medical students' exposure to violence: Impact on well being and perceived capacity to help battered women. *Journal of Comparative Family Studies, 34,* 113–135.

Ambuel, B., Hamberger, L. K., & Lahti, J. (1997). The Family Peace Project: A model for training healthcare professionals to identify, treat, and prevent partner violence. In L. K. Hamberger, S. Burge, A. Graham, & A. Costa (Eds.), *Violence issues for healthcare educators and providers* (pp. 55–81). Binghamton, NY: Haworth.

Bolin, L., & Elliott, B. A. (1996). Physician detection of family violence: Do buttons worn by doctors generate conversations about domestic violence? *Minnesota Medicine, 79,* 42–45.

Brown, J. B., Lent, B., & Sas, G. (1993). Identifying and treating wife abuse. *Journal of Family Practice, 36,* 185–191.

Dutton, D. G., & Painter, S. L. (1993). Emotional attachments in abusive relationships: A test of traumatic bonding theory. *Violence and Victims, 8,* 105–120.

Fletcher, J. L. (1994). "Medicalization" of America: Physician heal thy society? *American Family Physician, 49,* 1995.

Gazmararian, J. A., Lazorick, S., Spitz, A. M., Ballard, T. J., Saltzman, L. E., & Marks, J. S. (1996). Prevalence of violence against women. *Journal of the American Medical Association, 275,* 1915–1920.

Gerbert, B., Abercrombie, P., Caspers, P., Love, C., & Bronstone, A. (1999). How healthcare providers help battered women: The survivor's perspective. *Women and Health, 29,* 115–135.

Gerbert, B., Johnston, K., Caspers, N., Bleecker, T., Woods, A., & Rosenbaum, A. (1996). Experiences of battered women in healthcare settings: A qualitative study. *Women and Health, 24,* 1–17.

Hamberger, L. K., Ambuel, B., Marbella, A., & Donze, J. (1998). Physician interaction with battered women: The women's perspective. *Archives of Family Medicine, 7,* 575–582.

Hamberger, L. K., Guse, C., Boerger, J., Minsky, D., Pape, D., & Folsom, C. (in press). Evaluation of a healthcare provider training program to identify and help partner violence victims. *Journal of Family Violence.*

Hansen, M., Harway, M., & Cervantes, N. (1991). Therapists' perceptions of severity in cases of family violence. *Violence and Victims, 6*, 225–235.

Harwell, T. S., Casten, R. J., Armstrong, K. A., Dempsey, S., Coons, H. L., & Davis, M. (1998). Results of a domestic violence-training program offered to the staff of urban community health centers. *American Journal of Preventive Medicine, 15*, 235–242.

Hendricks-Matthews, M. K. (1991). A survey on violence education: A report of the STFM Violence Education Task Force. *Family Medicine, 23*, 194–197.

Kurz, D. (1987). Emergency department responses to battered women: Resistance to medicalization. *Social Problems, 34*, 69–81.

Larkin, G. L., Hyman, K. B., Mathias, S. R., D'Amico, F. D., & MacLeod, B. A. (1999). Universal screening for intimate partner violence in the emergency department: Importance of patient and provider factors. *Annals of Emergency Medicine, 33*, 669–675.

Larkin, G. L., Rolniak, S., Hyman, K. B., MacLeod, B. A., & Savage, R. (2000). Effects of an administrative intervention on rates of screening for domestic violence in an urban emergency department. *American Journal of Public Health, 90*, 1444–1448.

McGrath, M. E., Bettacchi, A., Duffy, S. J., Peipert, J. F., Becker, B. M., & St. Angelo, L. (1997). Violence against women: Provider barriers to intervention in emergency departments. *Academic Emergency Medicine, 4*, 297–300.

McLeer, S. V., Anwar, R. A., Herman, S., & Maquiling, K. (1989). Education is not enough: A system failure in protecting battered women. *Annals of Emergency Medicine, 18*, 651–653.

McNutt, L., Carlson, B. E., Gagen, D., & Winterbauer, N. (1999). Reproductive violence screening in primary care: Perspectives and experiences of patients and battered women. *Journal of the American Medical Women's Association, 54*, 85–90.

Melzer-Lange, M., Phelan, M. B., Hamberger, L. K., & Ambuel, B. (2000, September). *Current level of family violence education for one Midwestern medical school.* Paper presented at the 5th International Family Violence Conference, San Diego, CA.

Miles, A. (2000). *Domestic violence: What every pastor needs to know.* Minneapolis, MN: Fortress.

Minsky, D., Pape, D., & Hamberger, L. K. (2000, August). *Domestic violence: Qualitative analysis of barriers to identification and referral of victims in an urban healthcare setting.* Paper presented at the 108th Annual Convention of the American Psychological Association, Washington, DC.

Moore, M. L., Zaccaro, D., & Parsons, L. H. (1998). Attitudes and practices of nurses toward women who have experienced abuse/domestic violence. *Journal of Obstetric, Gynecologic and Neonatal Nursing, 27*, 175–182.

Olson, L., Anctil, C., Fullerton, L., Brillman, J., Arbuckle, J., & Sklar, D. (1996). Increasing emergency physician recognition of domestic violence. *Annals of Emergency Medicine, 27*, 741–746.

Panagiota, V. C., & Musialowski, R. (1997). Women's experiences with domestic violence and their attitudes and expectations regarding medical care of abuse victims. *Southern Medical Journal, 9,* 1075–1080.

Pape, D., Minsky, D., & Hamberger, L. K. (2000, August). *Hospital domestic violence initiatives: A long, bumpy, but worthwhile trip.* Paper presented at the 108th Annual Convention of the American Psychological Association, Washington, DC.

Patel, D., Hamberger, L. K., & Griffin, E. (2001, September). *Additive impact of training and a written protocol for screening and documentation of domestic violence by family physicians.* Paper presented at the meeting of the Nursing Network on Violence Against Women International, Madison, WI.

Phelan, M. B., Melzer-Lange, M., Hamberger, L. K., & Ambuel, B. (2000, September). *Current level of family violence education in residency programs of one Midwestern medical school.* Paper presented at the 5th International Family Violence Conference, San Diego, CA.

Plichta, S. B., Duncan, M. M., & Plichta, L. (1996). Spouse abuse, patient–physician communication, and patient satisfaction. *American Journal of Preventive Medicine, 12,* 297–303.

Roberts, G. L., Lawrence, J. M., O'Toole, B. I., & Raphael, B. (1997). Domestic violence in the emergency department: Detection by doctors and nurses. *General Hospital Psychiatry, 19,* 12–15.

Rodriguez, M. A., Bauer, H. M., McLoughlin, E., & Grumbach, K. (1999). Screening and intervention for intimate partner abuse: Practices and attitudes of primary care physicians. *Journal of the American Medical Association, 282,* 468–474.

Rodriguez, M. A., Craig, A. M., Mooney, D. R., & Bauer, H. M. (1998). Patient attitudes about mandatory reporting of domestic violence: Implications for healthcare professionals. *Western Journal of Medicine, 169,* 337–341.

Short, L. M., Cotton, D., & Hodgson, C. S. (1997). Evaluation of the module on domestic violence at the UCLA School of Medicine. *Academic Medicine, 72,* 75–92.

Stark, E., & Flitcraft, A. (1996). *Women at risk: Domestic violence and women's health.* Thousand Oaks, CA: Sage.

Stark, E., Flitcraft, A., Zuckerman, A., Grey, A., Robison, J., & Frazier, W. (1981). *Domestic violence: Wife abuse in the medical setting.* (Domestic violence monograph series No. 7). Washington, DC: National Clearinghouse on Domestic Violence.

Sugg, N. K., & Inui, T. (1992). Primary care physicians' response to domestic violence. *Journal of the American Medical Association, 267,* 3157–3160.

Thompson, R. S., Rivara, F. P., Thompson, D. C., Barlow, W. E., Sugg, N. K., Maiuro, R. D., & Rubanowice, D. M. (2000). Identification and management of domestic violence: A randomized trial. *American Journal of Preventive Medicine, 19,* 253–263.

Waalen, J., Goodwin, M. M., Spitz, A. M., Petersen, R., & Saltzman, L. E. (2000). Screening for intimate partner violence by healthcare providers: Barriers and interventions. *American Journal of Preventive Medicine, 19,* 230–237.

Warshaw, C. (1989). Limitations of the medical model in the care of battered women. *Gender and Society, 3,* 506–517.

5

ADVERSE CHILDHOOD EXPERIENCES AND HEALTH-RELATED QUALITY OF LIFE AS AN ADULT

VALERIE J. EDWARDS, ROBERT F. ANDA, VINCENT J. FELITTI, AND SHANTA R. DUBE

Domestic violence is only one type of family violence that leads people to seek medical care. Adult survivors of childhood abuse also often present in health care settings. Past abuse can lead to a number of health difficulties, and the more types of abuse patients experience, the greater the negative impact on health. This chapter presents new data on the health effects of multiple types of abuse and offers suggestions for providers on how to screen for and address the full range of traumatic events patients might have experienced.

Although medical histories are a staple of practice, most health care providers avoid asking adult patients about adverse childhood experiences (ACEs) such as abuse, neglect, exposure to intimate partner violence, and other forms of family dysfunction in the clinical setting. Not only are practitioners often unaware of the relevance of these experiences to adult health, but also they often believe such questions are invasive, threatening, and may interfere with the normal flow of care by causing emotional reactions in their patients. The omission of this crucial personal information in clinical practice is a serious shortcoming in current medical practice given that trauma underlies many persistent psychological conditions (G. Brown & Anderson, 1991), results in higher symptomatology and medical use (McCauley et al., 1997; Walker et al., 1999), and may interfere with adherence to medical regimens (Springs & Friedrich, 1992; Edwards, Anda, Gu, & Felitti, 2000).

Why should physicians and other medical practitioners care about childhood trauma experienced by their adult patients? First, it is not a rare phenomenon but rather represents a widespread problem in U.S. society. Prevalence estimates of childhood sexual abuse range from 15% to 28% in women and 5% to 15% in men (Finkelhor, 1994), and physical abuse is reported by approximately 25% of adults overall (MacMillan et al., 1997). Over 20% of adults report growing up with an alcoholic parent (Felitti et al., 1998). Despite these high prevalences, clinicians rarely consider that one in four women or one in five men they see were victimized as children.

Perhaps less widely known is the link between ACEs and chronic disease. Diabetes and the presence of diabetic symptoms have been linked to abuse both in childhood and later (Kendall-Tackett & Marshall, 1999). Our own research has demonstrated that ACEs underlie increased prevalences of the major causes of death and disability in the United States, including heart disease and cancer (Felitti et al., 1998). Other researchers have noted links between childhood abuse and both arthritis and breast cancer in women, as well as thyroid disease in men (Stein & Barrett-Connor, 2000).

Trauma also interferes with adherence to medical regimens and the effectiveness of health education interventions. People with ACEs are more likely to continue to smoke after diagnosis of conditions contraindicating smoking (Edwards et al., 2000). Adolescents and college-age women who were sexually abused as children have been shown to be at higher risk for HIV because of an impaired sense of self-efficacy about safe sex behavior (L. K. Brown, Kessel, Lourie, Ford, & Lipsitt, 1997; Johnsen & Harlow, 1996).

It is important to note that surveys have indicated that medical patients do not find questions about childhood trauma invasive or unwanted; rather, they overwhelmingly tend to endorse such inquiries and in fact generally believe that doctors and other health care professionals can help people cope with the aftereffects of abuse (Friedman, Samet, Roberts, Hudlin, & Hans, 1992). When we conducted the ACE Study (Felitti et al., 1998) in which we asked for sensitive information about childhood maltreatment and family dysfunction, a 24-hr staffed phone line for patients potentially distressed by survey questions received no calls from more than 30,000 recipients. In addition, there was little noncompliance with answering questions about child abuse, as less than 7% of more than 18,000 respondents did not respond to questions on sexual abuse.

WHY ASK ABOUT
MULTICATEGORY TRAUMA?

Earlier research in child maltreatment tended to focus on a single type of abuse (i.e., sexual abuse or physical abuse). As the field has evolved, there has been a growing understanding that children at risk for one type of maltreatment frequently experience other types. Evidence that a majority of people who report one type of trauma have experienced additional types has been gathered from such diverse samples as women in specialty medical care (Leserman, Li, Hu, & Drossman, 1998), female veterans (Read, Stern, Wolfe, & Ouimette, 1997), and psychiatric outpatients (Engels, Moisan, & Harris, 1994). These findings closely mirror the results of the ACE Study, in which the presence of one type of childhood abuse (physical, sexual, or emotional) was a strong indicator that other adverse childhood experiences had occurred (Anda et al., 1999; Felitti et al., 1998). For instance, in homes where children witness partner violence, physical abuse of the children, as well as alcohol or drug abuse, was often present (Dube et al., 2001). Therefore, it is likely that studies comparing people who have experienced one type of abuse with nonabused controls are actually composed of a more heterogeneous sample that may obscure group differences, thereby resulting in weaker abuse effects.

Moreover, trauma acts as a cumulative stressor. The strength of the relation between the experience and the outcome increases in a dose–response manner as more ACEs are reported. For example, reports from the ACE Study have found strong, graded associations between childhood maltreatment experiences and teen pregnancy (Dietz et al., 1999), male involvement in teen pregnancy (Anda, Chapman, et al., 2002), smoking (Anda et al., 1999), depression and alcoholism (Anda, Whitfield, et al., 2002), and sexually transmitted diseases (Hillis, Anda, Felitti, Nordenberg, & Marchbanks, 2000). Other researchers (Leserman et al., 1998; Moeller, Bachmann, & Moeller, 1993) have similarly reported rises in symptomatology and poor health status as the number of reported abuse categories increased. It is not surprising that Walker et al. (1999) noted that increases in the median annual health care costs of health maintenance organization members were related to the rise in the number of reported abuse types.

Furthermore, trauma changes developmental trajectories that in turn increase the probability of additional trauma risk (Cicchetti, Toth, & Maughan, 2000). For instance, women who have been sexually abused in childhood are at greater risk for assault in adulthood than those without an abusive background (Mandoki & Burkhart, 1989; Urquiza & Goodlin-Jones, 1994; Wyatt, Guthrie, & Notgrass, 1992).

WHY ASSESS THE OVERALL HEALTH EFFECTS OF ADVERSE CHILDHOOD EXPERIENCES?

Just as the study of the effects of ACEs has proceeded in a fragmented way, the health effects of victimization have been investigated as a collection of symptoms and various disease conditions without a unifying construct besides "poor health." This haphazard approach reflects the experience of clinicians in various subspecialties of medicine, each of whom have independently "discovered" that many of their patients report childhood abuse. However, these findings may not adequately capture the overall effects of childhood maltreatment on the more general aspects of health functioning. Rather than continuing to assess health outcomes in a piecemeal, syndrome-by-syndrome fashion, it is instead critical to consider the impact ACEs may have on health-related quality of life independent of specific disease conditions. We were able to assess this in the second wave of the ACE Study by administering a measure of health-related quality of life to participants who had already completed a detailed background questionnaire on their childhood experiences.

METHOD

The Adverse Childhood Experiences Study

The ACE Study was undertaken to assess the effects of a broad range of negative childhood experiences on adult health behavior and medical conditions. Conducted at Kaiser Permanente's Health Appraisal Clinic (HAC) in San Diego, California, this is one of the largest studies of the prevalence of ACEs in a community sample.

Participants were health maintenance organization members undergoing a comprehensive medical evaluation; this approach allowed us to assess their current health condition in addition to their childhood history related to abuse and family dysfunction. Conducted in two survey waves, the ACE Study includes more than 18,000 participants between the ages of 19 and 90. More complete descriptions of the study procedures have been published previously (Anda et al., 2000; Felitti et al., 1998). The data presented here are derived from the second survey wave, conducted between June and October of 1997. In the first survey wave, 70.5% of respondents completed the instrument, and 65% (8,667/13,300) returned a completed ACE questionnaire in the second wave, for an overall response rate of 68%. Analyses on the first-wave participants (Edwards et al., 2001) indicate that demographic differences between responders and nonresponders were similar to those found in survey research: Nonresponders were younger, less educated, and from racial–ethnic minority groups. After controlling for these demographic differences, however, no evidence of significant differences in the overall health status of responders and nonresponders was found.

Instruments

Family health history. The Family Health History is a 168-item questionnaire that was mailed to members' homes prior to their visit to the HAC. It covers a broad range of childhood exposures and current health behaviors. Information about ACEs was derived from responses to this questionnaire. Specifically, we coded for the presence of any of the following eight ACEs: (a) physical abuse, (b) sexual abuse, (c) verbal abuse, (d) witnessing maternal battering, (e) growing up with an alcoholic or drug-abusing family member, (f) growing up with a family member who was put in prison, (g) having parents who were separated or divorced, and (h) growing up with a family member who was depressed or mentally ill. We totaled the number of categories of reported ACEs (range: 0–8) and then collapsed the upper end of the range (4 or higher) to create an ordinal measure with five levels (0, 1, 2, 3, 4 or more ACEs).

Medical Outcome Study Short-Form 36-Item Health Survey (SF-36). The SF-36 questionnaire (Ware & Sherbourne, 1992) is a widely used instrument that measures the extent to which one's physical or mental health is a limiting factor in the enjoyment of life. The survey consists of eight subscales; results from seven of these are presented here: (a) Physical Functioning, a measure of the extent to which one can perform normal life activities; (b) Role–Physical, a measure of how much work or other daily activities are affected by physical health; (c) Bodily Pain, a measure of the extent to which somatic symptoms interfere with the enjoyment of life; (d) General Health, which measures a person's overall assessment of the state of his or her health; (e) Vitality, a measure of one's energy and activity; (f) Social Functioning, a measure of how much one's physical or emotional problems interfere with social activities; and (g) Role–Emotional, a measure of the extent to which emotional problems interfere with work or other activities. Higher scores indicate better functioning on each health dimension. Scale norms for men and women by age allow investigators to compare the findings in their sample to a broader population. We collected SF-36 data in the second survey wave by asking HAC patients to complete the questionnaire in the waiting room before their physical examination. Thus, 7,641 of the 8,667 (88.2%) study participants are included in these analyses.

Analyses

Separate analyses for men and women were performed to facilitate comparison with available SF-36 norms. Linear regression analyses on the

SF-36 subscales were conducted controlling for age using ACE score as an ordinal independent variable.

RESULTS

Description of the Sample

The average age of the participants was 56.0 (SD = 15.04). The sample was overwhelmingly White (74.4%); Hispanics (10.3%) and Asian/Pacific Islanders (7.0%) were the largest minority groups represented. Over three quarters (77.5%) of the respondents had at least some college or a college degree.

Prevalence of Adverse Childhood Experiences

The prevalence of each of the individual ACEs used to compute the ACE score is listed by gender in Table 5.1. Men reported statistically more physical abuse than women. There were no differences by gender in reports of violent treatment of one's mother. Women reported significantly more sexual abuse, emotional abuse, household substance abuse and mental illness, prison time by a family member, and separation or divorce of parents.

The numbers and percentages of respondents for each level of the ACE score is listed by gender in Table 5.2. It is interesting that over 38% (N = 3,317) of all respondents reported two or more ACEs in their childhood; 12.9% (N = 1,115) reported four or more ACEs. Consistent with the finding that women reported more individual ACEs, more women than men were represented at each level of the ACE score, $\chi^2(4, N = 7641) = 55.67$, $p < .0001$.

TABLE 5.1
Prevalence of Individual Adverse Childhood Experiences (ACEs) by Gender

	Men		Women		Total		
ACE	N	%	N	%	N	%	χ^2
Physical abuse	992	28.3	1,010	24.5	2,002	26.2	14.16**
Sexual abuse	581	17.0	981	24.6	1,562	21.1	64.61*
Emotional abuse	298	8.2	480	11.6	767	10.0	24.98*
Family mental illness/suicide	504	14.4	1,023	24.8	1,527	20.0	128.74*
Family substance abuse	883	25.1	1,229	29.8	2,112	27.6	20.15*
Violent treatment of mother	421	12.2	556	13.5	997	12.9	2.74
Family member in prison	170	4.9	284	6.9	454	6.0	14.18*
Parental separation/divorce	785	22.5	1,032	25.2	1,817	24.0	7.07*

*p < .001. **p < .0001. $\chi^2(1, N = 7641)$.

TABLE 5.2
Prevalence of Adverse Childhood Experience (ACE) Score by Gender

ACE score	Men N	Men %	Women N	Women %	Total N	Total %
0	1,331	37.9	1,425	34.5	2,756	36.1
1	966	27.5	1,063	25.1	2,002	26.2
2	567	16.1	641	15.5	1,208	15.8
3	309	8.8	414	10.0	723	9.5
4 or more	338	9.6	614	14.9	952	12.5

Health-Related Quality of Life

Consistent with SF-36 norms (Ware & Sherbourne, 1992), men had statistically higher mean scores on each scale than women (see Table 5.3). Each of the overall age-adjusted scale means for men and women were within one standard deviation of the national norm. Table 5.4 illustrates the impact of the ACE score on self-perceptions of health, after adjustment for age. For each health dimension, there were strong, linear decrements in each scale as exposure to different types of childhood maltreatment and family dysfunction (ACE score) increased, with some variation in this response by gender. Among men, there were very small differences in scale scores between an ACE score of 2 and 3, but there was a drop in scale scores between an ACE score of 3 and 4. Overall, women's SF-36 scores showed a stronger dose–response relationship between the ACE score and each of the scales than did men's scale scores. However, a multivariate analysis of variance to test the Gender × ACE score interaction was not significant for any of the scales. Of all the SF-36 dimensions, the Bodily Pain scale showed the largest negative change, and respondents with four or more ACEs scored one standard deviation lower than the national norm.

TABLE 5.3
Mean SF-36 Scale Scores by Gender

SF-36 Scale	Men	Women	Total
Physical Functioning**	84.49	79.60	81.86
Role–Physical**	82.18	76.78	79.27
Bodily Pain**	73.41	69.28	71.19
General Health*	75.59	74.75	75.14
Vitality**	64.38	59.10	61.55
Social Functioning**	89.00	85.73	87.25
Role–Emotional**	89.11	84.00	86.50

*p < .039. **p < .0001.

TABLE 5.4
Age-Adjusted SF-36 Scale Means by Adverse Childhood Experience (ACE) Score and Gender

ACE score	Physical Functioning		Role–Physical		Bodily Pain		General Health		Vitality		Social Functioning		Role–Emotional	
	Men	Women	Men	Women	Men	Women	Men	Women	Men	Women	Men	Women	Men	Women
0	86.52	82.99	87.16	81.86	77.17	73.48	77.44	76.66	67.07	63.17	92.53	89.41	93.02	88.53
1	86.18	81.00	83.98	78.43	75.25	70.15	76.60	76.04	66.15	60.37	90.18	87.87	90.68	85.44
2	84.08	80.16	80.67	78.13	70.63	70.56	75.14	75.80	62.76	59.19	87.21	86.37	86.88	84.84
3	84.10	78.07	79.64	73.90	70.29	67.98	75.54	74.28	63.81	57.23	88.67	84.82	88.04	82.33
4 or more	81.93	77.56	76.55	71.51	68.61	64.26	72.24	72.39	59.43	54.81	83.91	80.39	83.21	77.45
Total	85.93	80.21	84.16	77.46	74.32	70.06	76.21	75.43	65.01	60.03	89.78	86.76	90.08	84.78

DISCUSSION

Traumatic experiences decades earlier exerted a powerful influence on perceptions of current well-being across a range of health dimensions. How these experiences translate into particular health problems may be due to the confluence of genetic and environmental influences on specific physical systems. Rather than expecting that ACEs would translate into particular medical conditions, it seems more likely that they would exert a pernicious influence across the full spectrum of physiological and mental functioning. Given that previous research has established that self-ratings of health are strongly related to clinical measures (Mansson & Rastam, 2001; Long & Marshall, 1999), it is likely that SF-36 ratings are accurate self-assessments of current health functioning.

These results echo and amplify previous findings in the area of health and childhood maltreatment (Briere, 1992; Golding, 1999; Moeller et al., 1993). In particular, large decrements in the Bodily Pain scale, a measure of somatization, were seen. The inclusion of men in this analysis is of critical importance, because little information on the effects of victimization on men's health has been previously available. Results from this study indicate that maltreatment produced comparable decrements in men's and women's SF-36 scale scores.

Treating Victims of Multiple Abuse

Although screening is a prerequisite to treating the effects of multiple abuse, most often the patient's history of childhood adversity is at present considered to be outside the scope of routine medical visits. Without screening, practitioners often find themselves chasing an unrelated set of symptoms with no evident unifying medical condition. We do not mean to imply that illness in victims of ACEs is solely stress related; rather, it appears that the psychic distress associated with ACEs can underlie a diverse set of conditions, including organic diseases. Although it is vitally important that practitioners do not assume that the presence of ACEs are the root of a patient's problems, it is equally important that the high prevalence of ACEs not be avoided and missed in routine medical practice. Helping the patient to explore the role ACEs may play in his or her current health functioning is critical, because the link is powerful—even after many years have passed.

Although psychotherapy is the traditional choice, we believe that a wide variety of therapeutic modalities should be available to best treat people who report multiple ACEs. At Kaiser Permanente's Positive Choice Wellness Center in San Diego, patients may participate in theater workshops, movement therapy, and expressive-writing and diary programs as adjuncts to or instead of traditional psychotherapeutic interventions. In addition, referrals for hypnotherapy are available.

Expressive-writing techniques, such as those used by Pennebaker and his colleagues (Pennebaker, Kiecolt-Glaser, & Glaser, 1988; Petrie, Booth, & Pennebaker, 1995), have been found to be useful in reducing symptoms across a wide range of conditions. A recent meta-analysis concluded that expressive-writing techniques can improve physical and psychological well-being as well as physical functioning (Smyth, 1998). Theater techniques have been invaluable, because they often enable people to speak about the unspeakable by using archetypes to role play life experiences (Eulert, 1998). Hypnosis is not a treatment per se but a framework in which treatment can be carried out more efficiently (we are referring here to Ericksonian, not "command," hypnosis). Many patients are skeptical of the benefits of hypnotherapy, but dramatic results can often be achieved. One patient, who was suicidal after substantial weight loss had caused long-standing issues stemming from multiple maltreatment to re-emerge, agreed to see a hypnotherapist, thinking, "I'll be polite before I die." She left the hypnotherapy session relieved of suicidal ideation and with a set of tools she refers to as "invaluable" (Alman, 2001).

Recommendations for Changing Medical Practice

We believe that universal screening for a wide variety of ACEs, such as those measured by the ACE Study, should be considered a part of routine medical care. This could be accomplished most efficiently by including questions on ACEs in a general medical history completed by patients before their medical examinations. We have found that most patients answer these inquiries candidly and that few object to their inclusion. The availability of brief, effective questionnaires, as well as the potential utility of such screening in curbing medical costs, may bring this practice into greater use.

However, research indicates that many medical practitioners find this information on ACEs personally threatening (Ronnberg & Hammarstrom, 2000) and are therefore reluctant to talk to their patients about these experiences. In addition, many clinicians feel ill equipped to deal with the responsibility of this information and fear that they may cause their patients further upset (Sugg & Inui, 1992). We believe that the most important follow-up question a medical practitioner can ask when a patient reports childhood trauma, is "How has that experience affected you in your adult life?" This simple question can provide a window into the cause of poor health functioning in affected patients.

Even when a practitioner is willing to discuss childhood trauma with his or her adult patients, it is imperative that appropriate referrals are available. Better coordination of mental and physical health services, and greater insurance coverage for both traditional and nontraditional therapies, would greatly enhance the confidence with which medical practitioners may enter into these important discussions with their patients. Furthermore, additional research is needed to assess the efficacy of various therapeutic modalities to assure that the most effective treatments are available to these patients.

Finally, much more needs to be done so that the links between childhood maltreatment and poor adult health can be better understood. Future studies should explore potential intervention points, such as weight control, smoking cessation, and alcohol and drug programs, that may benefit by considering the connection between ACEs and the adoption and maintenance of poor health behaviors. This may, in turn, lead to the development of more effective interventions to treat these conditions among people with ACEs. Without better understanding of the critical interaction, the legacy of ACEs will continue to affect millions of victims, at a great cost to themselves and to society in terms of poor health.

REFERENCES

Alman, B. (2001). Medical hypnosis: An underutilized treatment approach. *The Permanente Journal, 5,* 35–39.

Anda, R. F., Chapman, D. P., Felitti, V. J., Edwards, V. J., Williamson, D. F., Croft, J. B., & Giles, W. H. (2002). Adverse childhood experiences and risk of paternity in teen pregnancy. *Obstetrics and Gynecology, 100,* 37–45.

Anda, R. F., Croft, J. B., Felitti, V. J., Nordenberg, D., Giles, W. H., Williamson, D. F., & Giovino, G. A. (1999). Adverse childhood experiences and smoking during adolescence and adulthood. *Journal of the American Medical Association, 282,* 1652–1658.

Anda, R. F., Whitfield, C. L., Felitti, V. J., Chapman, D., Edwards, V. J., Dube, S. R., & Williamson, D. F. (2002). Alcohol-impaired parents and adverse childhood experiences: The risk of depression and alcoholism during adulthood. *Journal of Psychiatric Services, 53,* 1001–1009.

Briere, J. (1992). Medical symptoms, health risk, and history of childhood sexual abuse. *Mayo Clinic Proceedings, 67,* 603–604.

Brown, G., & Anderson, B. (1991). Psychiatric morbidity in adult inpatients with childhood histories of sexual and physical abuse. *American Journal of Psychiatry, 148,* 55–61.

Brown, L. K., Kessel, S. M., Lourie, K. J., Ford, H. H., & Lipsitt, L. P. (1997). Influence of sexual abuse on HIV-related attitudes and behaviors in adolescent psychiatric inpatients. *Journal of the American Academy of Child and Adolescent Psychiatry, 36,* 316–322.

Cicchetti, D., Toth, S. L., & Maughan, A. (2000). An ecological–transactional model of child maltreatment. In A. J. Sameroff et al. (Eds.), *Handbook of developmental psychopathology* (2nd ed., pp. 689–722). New York: Kluwer Academic/Plenum.

Dietz, P. M., Spitz, A. M., Anda, R. F., Williamson, D. F., McMahon, P. M., Santelli, J. S., et al. (1999). Unintended pregnancy among adult women exposed to abuse or household dysfunction during their childhood. *Journal of the American Medical Society, 282,* 1359–1364.

Dube, S. R., Anda, R. F., Felitti, V. J., Croft, J. B., Edwards, V. J., & Giles, W. H. (2001). Growing up with parental alcohol abuse: Exposure to childhood abuse, neglect, and household dysfunction. *Child Abuse and Neglect, 25,* 1627–1640.

Edwards, V. J., Anda, R. F., Gu, D., & Felitti, V. J. (November, 2000). *The relation between childhood abuse and smoking persistence in adults with smoking-related symptoms and diseases.* Paper presented at the 14th National Chronic Disease conference, Dallas, TX.

Edwards, V. J., Anda, R. F., Nordenberg, D. F., Felitti, V. J., Williamson, D. F., Howard, N., & Wright, J. A. (2001). Factors affecting probability of response to a survey about childhood abuse. *Child Abuse and Neglect, 25,* 307–312.

Engels, M., Moisan, D., & Harris, R. (1994). MMPI indices of childhood trauma among 110 female outpatients. *Journal of Personality Assessment, 63,* 135–147.

Eulert, C. H. (1998). *The magic chest: Where you are, where you've been, where you're going?* Washington, DC: Taylor & Francis.

Felitti, V. J., Anda, R. F., Nordenberg, D., Williamson, D. F., Spitz, A. M., Edwards, V., et al. (1998). Relationship of child abuse and household dysfunction to many of the leading causes of death in adults. *American Journal of Preventive Medicine, 14,* 245–258.

Finkelhor, D. (1994). Current information on the scope and nature of child sexual abuse. *Future of Children, 4,* 31–53.

Friedman, L. S., Samet, J. H., Roberts, M. S., Hudlin, M., & Hans, P. (1992). Inquiry about victimization experiences: A survey of patient preferences and physician practices. *Archives of Internal Medicine, 152,* 1186–1190.

Golding, J. M. (1999). Sexual-assault history and long-term physical health problems: Evidence from clinical and population epidemiology. *Current Directions in Psychological Science, 8,* 191–194.

Hillis, S. D., Anda, R. F., Felitti, V. J., Nordenberg, D., & Marchbanks, P. (2000). Adverse childhood experiences and sexually transmitted diseases in men and women: A retrospective study. *Pediatrics, 106,* E11.

Johnsen, L. W., & Harlow, L. L. (1996). Childhood sexual abuse linked with adult substance abuse, victimization, and AIDS-risk. *AIDS Education and Prevention, 8,* 44–57.

Kendall-Tackett, K., & Marshall, R. (1999). Victimization and diabetes: An exploratory study. *Child Abuse and Neglect, 23,* 593–596.

Leserman, J., Li, Z., Hu, J. B., & Drossman, D. A. (1998). How multiple types of stressors impact on health. *Psychosomatic Medicine, 60,* 175–181.

Long, M. J., & Marshall, B. S. (1999). The relationship between self-assessed health status, mortality, service use, and cost in a managed care setting. *Health Care Management Review, 24,* 20–27.

MacMillan, H. L., Fleming, J. E., Trocme, N., Boyle, M. H., Wong, M., Racine, Y. A., et al. (1997). Prevalence of child physical and sexual abuse in the community: Results from the Ontario Health Supplement. *Journal of the American Medical Association, 278,* 131–135.

Mandoki, C. A., & Burkhart, B. R. (1989). Sexual victimization: Is there a vicious cycle? *Violence and Victims, 4,* 179–190.

Mansson, N. O., & Rastam, L. (2001). Self-rated health as a predictor of disability pension and death: A prospective study of middle-aged men. *Scandinavian Journal of Public Health, 29,* 151–158.

McCauley, J., Kern, D. E., Kolodner, K., Dill, L., Schroeder, A. F., DeChant, H. K., et al. (1997). Clinical characteristics of women with a history of childhood abuse: Unhealed wounds. *Journal of the American Medical Association, 277,* 1362–1368.

Moeller, T. P., Bachmann, G. A., & Moeller, J. A. (1993). The combined effects of physical, sexual, and emotional abuse during childhood: Long-term health consequences for women. *Child Abuse and Neglect, 17,* 623–640.

Pennebaker, J. W., Kiecolt-Glaser, J., & Glaser, R. (1988). Disclosure of traumas and immune function: Health implications for psychotherapy. *Journal of Consulting and Clinical Psychology, 56,* 239–245.

Petrie, K., Booth, R., & Pennebaker, J. (1995). Disclosure of trauma and immune response to a hepatitis B vaccination program. *Journal of Consulting and Clinical Psychology, 6,* 787–792.

Read, J. P, Stern, A. L., Wolfe, J., & Ouimette, P. C. (1997). Use of a screening instrument in women's health care: Detecting relationships among victimization history, psychological distress, and medical complaints. *Women and Health, 25,* 1–17.

Ronnberg, A. K., & Hammarstrom, A. (2000). Barriers within the health care system to dealing with sexualized violence: A literature review. *Scandinavian Journal of Public Health, 28,* 222–229.

Smyth, J. M. (1998). Written emotional expression: Effect sizes, outcome types, and moderating variables. *Journal of Consulting and Clinical Psychology, 66,* 174–184.

Springs, F., & Friedrich, W. N. (1992). Health risk behaviors and medical sequelae of childhood sexual abuse. *Mayo Clinic Proceedings, 67,* 527–532.

Stein, M. B., & Barrett-Connor, E. (2000). Sexual assault and physical health: Findings from a population-based study of older adults. *Psychosomatic Medicine, 62,* 838–843.

Sugg, N. K., & Inui, T. (1992). Primary care physicians' response to domestic violence. Opening Pandora's box. *Journal of the American Medical Association, 267,* 3157–3160.

Urquiza, A. J., & Goodlin-Jones, B. L. (1994). Child sexual abuse and adult revictimization with women of color. *Violence and Victims, 9*, 223–232.

Walker, E. A., Unutzer, J., Rutter, C., Gelfand, A., Saunders, K., VonKorff, M., et al. (1999). Costs of health care use by women HMO members with a history of childhood abuse and neglect. *Archives of General Psychiatry, 56*, 609–613.

Ware, J. E., & Sherbourne, C. D. (1992). The MOS 36-Item Short-Form Health Survey (SF-36): I. Conceptual framework and item selection. *Medical Care, 30*, 473–483.

Wyatt, G. E., Guthrie, D., & Notgrass, C. M. (1992). Differential effects of women's child sexual abuse and subsequent sexual revictimization. *Journal of Consulting and Clinical Psychology, 60*, 167–173.

6

VICTIMIZATION OF CHILDREN WITH DISABILITIES

LIZA LITTLE

Recent research has revealed that children with disabilities are a distinct high-risk group for victimization and maltreatment, being on average two to three times more likely to be abused. Abused children with disabilities often present in health care settings, but abuse may be masked by their condition. In this chapter, some of the unique vulnerabilities of children with disabilities are described. Adults who had disabilities as children should also be screened for past and current abuse. Disabled adults are susceptible to all the health effects that nondisabled adults face. In addition, abuse can add to and strengthen the impact of their disability. Suggestions are offered for assessment, reporting, and treatment of victimization in this population.

Children with disabilities are one of society's most vulnerable populations (Ammerman, 1997; National Center on Child Abuse and Neglect, 1993; Sullivan & Knutson, 2000). There is a dearth of research on the maltreatment of children with disabilities, and even basic investigative data collection procedures of maltreated children often fail to record whether a child has a disability. Only 19 states in the United States require that disability status be recorded when a complaint of child maltreatment is made (National Clearinghouse on Child Abuse and Neglect Information, 2001). Overt and covert attitudinal barriers by clinicians toward individuals

95

with disabilities may affect the accessibility, availability, and adaptability of treatment (Mansell, Sobsey, & Moskal, 1998). Indeed, the extensive fields of family violence and child maltreatment research have focused minimally on the victimization of children with disabilities. The belief that developmentally delayed children, for instance, cannot benefit from psychotherapy, or that they are somehow less affected by abuse, or less interesting to work with, can undermine the quality of the assessment and treatment a child with disabilities receives (Mansell et al., 1998).

In this chapter I discuss the prevalence rates for maltreatment of children with disabilities, the relationship between disability and victimization, and the risk factors for victimization for children with disabilities. I apply an ecological framework to address assessment and treatment issues.

PREVALENCE OF MALTREATMENT OF CHILDREN WITH DISABILITIES

There is an enormous range and heterogeneity of disabilities that can afflict children. The most common forms include learning disabilities, behavior disorders, and mental retardation (Sullivan & Knutson, 1998). Seventy-one percent of all children with disabilities fall into these categories. There is considerable evidence that disabilities are a risk factor for maltreatment.

Data from the second National Incidence Study of Child Abuse and Neglect indicate that approximately 21.3 per 1,000 children without disabilities are maltreated each year, compared with 35.5 per 1,000 children with disabilities. In other words, 175,000–300,000 U.S. children with disabilities are abused or neglected each year (National Clearinghouse on Child Abuse and Neglect Information, 2001; Westat Inc., 1993). The study authors concluded that children with disabilities were 1.7 times more likely to be maltreated than children without disabilities. Sullivan and Knutson (1998) estimated that these figures are probably low, because child protective services workers were asked to make the diagnosis of disability, and they are generally not qualified to do so. Moreover, these findings do not include extrafamilial abuse, because information about abuse outside the family is in police records rather than in state child protective services records.

Embry (2001) conducted a retrospective study of 770 deaf adults who were also deaf as children. Forty-five percent of the sample reported some type of abuse, 19% reported caregiver physical abuse, 30% reported residential staff physical abuse, 18% reported sexual abuse, and 9% reported physical neglect. Of interest is that parent communication method did not predict any type of maltreatment; however, poor communication between parents and children increased the risk of neglect, and fair communication quality increased the risk for caregiver physical abuse.

From a methodological standpoint, Sullivan and Knutson's (2000) recent study of 50,278 young and school-age children is perhaps the best. The sample comprised children who were enrolled in the public and parochial schools in Omaha, Nebraska, for grades K–12. The sample also included children who were eligible for special education and early intervention programs (e.g., Zero to Three, Early Intervention Preschool). Therefore, the ages ranged from 0 to 21. The sample was 51.4% male and 48.6% female. The ethnicity of the sample was 67% Caucasian, 25% African American, 5% Hispanic, and 3% Asian American or Native American.

Among the 3,262 children with identified disabilities, the types of disability were as follows: behavioral disorders (37.4%), mental retardation (25.3%), learning disabled (16.4%), health related (11.2%), speech/language (6.5%), physical/orthopedic disabilities (1.2%), hearing impairment (1.3%), visual impairment (0.4%), and autism (0.1%). These categories were collapsed as follows: behavior (behavior disorders and autism); communication disorders (speech, language, hearing, and learning disabilities); mental retardation (all levels—mild to profound); and orthopedic and health related (visual impairment; orthopedic disabilities; and health-related disabilities, including asthma and juvenile rheumatoid arthritis). Approximately 13% of these children's disabilities were due to health problems.

Sullivan and Knutson (2000) identified 4,503 maltreated children, 1,012 of whom also had an identified disability. The overall rate of maltreatment for children without disabilities was 11%. For children with disabilities, the overall rate was 31%. The authors found that children with disabilities were 3.4 times more likely to be neglected and physically, emotionally, or sexually abused compared with children who did not have disabilities.

Children with disabilities are two to three times more likely to be abused or neglected in their homes and to be victims of family violence than are nondisabled children (National Center on Child Abuse and Neglect, 1993; Sullivan & Knutson, 1998, 2000). In other studies, children with disabilities who are living in institutional settings and residential homes are two to four times more likely to be sexually abused than children without disabilities (Ammerman, 1997; Sobsey, Randall, & Parrila, 1997; Sullivan & Knutson, 1998).

Maltreatment of children with disabilities is not limited to homes or state institutions. Cognitively and physically disabled children are also at greater risk for peer victimization and exclusion in their school communities than are their nondisabled peers (Cook & Semmel, 1999; Little, 2002; Llewellyn, 1995; Morrison, Furlong, & Smith, 1994; Santich & Kavanagh, 1997; Thompson, Whitney, & Smith, 1994). In one national study on assault rates in communities, young, intellectually disabled men were found to be at greatest risk for assault (Coleman, 1997). Children with disabilities are also more likely to suffer multiple forms of maltreatment when they are abused than are children who are maltreated but do not have disabilities (Sullivan & Knutson, 2000). This fact alone has great implications for practitioners who work with children with disabilities and have experienced abuse and neglect; it suggests that assessment must be multiproblem focused.

RELATIONSHIP BETWEEN DISABILITY AND VICTIMIZATION

The cause-and-effect relationship between disability and maltreatment is complex, because physical trauma and environmental deprivation can cause a child to acquire a disability. Shaken baby syndrome, for instance, whereby whiplash injury to the brain occurs, may cause permanent physical and neurological damage to an infant (Mitchell & Buchele-Ash, 2000). Other evidence shows that child maltreatment is associated with the development of conduct disorders in children (Sullivan & Knutson, 1998). The question of whether it is the child's disability that provokes the maltreatment, the maltreatment that creates the disability, or the pervasive social and psychological intolerance by individuals in the child's social ecology that causes the maltreatment are all important areas for the clinician to explore (Mitchell & Buchele-Ash, 2000). Understanding that the relationship between disability and victimization is not unidirectional can help to decrease scripted thinking and bias about children with disabilities.

Explanations for the increased incidence of maltreatment of children with disabilities suggest that children with severe communication and behavioral disorders, or developmental delays, may create higher emotional, physical, and economic demands on parents that lead to greater parental and family stress, caregiver burden, and compassion fatigue (Committee on Child Abuse and Neglect and Committee on Children With Disabilities, 2001). Lack of respite care for parents caring for children with severe disabilities can also contribute to an increase in risk for child abuse and neglect (Committee on Child Abuse and Neglect and Committee on Children With Disabilities, 2001; Rodriguez & Murphy, 1997). In addition, if the child has difficultly with communication and has behavior problems, caregivers may be easily frustrated by the child's inability to respond to traditional means of discipline or behavioral reinforcement, which can increase the child's risk for maltreatment (Sullivan & Cork, 1998). These explanations are theoretical at best and require further empirical substantiation.

UNDERSTANDING ABUSE USING AN
ECOLOGICAL FRAMEWORK

The theoretical perspective adopted in considering the needs of mal-treated children with disabilities may shape the treatment and interventions chosen for any given child and can guide treatment decisions for adult survivors as well. The National Research Council on Children identified ecological theory as a framework best suited to address the causes, conse-quences, and treatment formulations for abused children (U.S. Department of Health and Human Services, 1997). The contextual contributions of the child's environment, and the potential interactions among different systems, are essential features of this model (Grauerholz, 2000).

In this model, maltreatment is multiply determined by factors operating at different levels of systems influencing the child. This includes the individ-ual child, the child's family, the community, and the culture at large (Belsky, 1993). These factors create the context for child abuse and are intertwined in a social ecology so that no factor alone is responsible for the etiology of the maltreatment (Belsky, 1993).

Nowhere is the ecological model more important than in the consider-ation of maltreated children with disabilities. This model helps to frame assessment and treatment in terms of multiple perspectives and is more likely to generate hypotheses, minimize overinterpretation, and prevent the focus on single causes or short-term effects or the exclusive focus on the individual child and his or her disability (Llewellyn & Hogan, 2000; Sullivan & Cork, 1998).

A child with a disability may be bullied at school, yelled at at home, shunned on the school bus, and be coping with multiple stressors that extend from interactions in his or her family to those with school peers, teachers, and the greater community. Parents of some children with disabilities may likewise be struggling: Addressing the various barriers to procuring services for their child; providing adequate care; getting respite breaks; and managing families, marriages, and jobs may overwhelm them. Teachers and school systems can also feel victimized by resource limitations, exclusionary regula-tions, and lack of training (Weinberg, 1997). Assessing the social context in which the abuse occurs is an important initial step to planning effec-tive treatment.

Children at Risk

There are many different types of disabilities. For research purposes, they are often grouped into categories that include behavioral, communica-tion, mental retardation, and health- and orthopedic-related disabilities. The most common form of maltreatment among children with disabilities is neglect, followed by physical, emotional, and sexual abuse (Sullivan & Knutson, 2000).

Sullivan and Knutson (2000) broke down the relative risk rates of maltreatment by types of disabilities and found the following results:

- Children with behavioral disorders are seven times more likely to be physically abused, emotionally abused, and neglected, and five times more likely to be sexually abused.
- Children with speech and language difficulties have five times the risk for neglect and physical abuse and three times the risk for sexual abuse.
- Children with developmental delays have four times the risk for neglect and physical, sexual, and emotional abuse.
- Children with hearing impairments have twice the risk for neglect and emotional abuse and almost four times the risk for physical abuse.

Younger children with disabilities are at higher risk for all forms of maltreatment. In terms of gender, boys with disabilities are at greater risk for physical abuse, and girls with disabilities are at greater risk for sexual abuse (Sobsey et al., 1997). Children with severe communication and intellectual deficits and language barriers are all at higher risk for victimization, because they may not be able to use language to express their needs and are therefore more vulnerable to abuse (Mansell et. al., 1998).

There are some newer areas of victimization, such as on-line victimization of children. Children using the Internet have been exposed to pornography and lured into sexual talk and virtual sex, and some actual encounters and kidnappings have taken place (Finkelhor, Mitchell, & Wolak, 2000). It is unclear whether children with disabilities are at greater risk for these occurrences, but many children with disabilities, particularly those with physical disabilities, those with mobility issues, and those who are homebound much of the time, often rely on the Internet for socialization and connection to the greater world. Expanding clinical screening to include questions concerning on-line victimization should now be included for all children, but especially for children with disabilities. This area clearly requires further study (Finkelhor et al., 2000).

Families at Risk

In general, the causes of abuse and neglect of children with disabilities are no different than those for all children (Committee on Child Abuse and Neglect and Committee on Children With Disabilities, 2001). Children with disabilities whose families have multiple risk factors, including poverty, domestic violence, drug and alcohol abuse, single-parent status, or unemployment, are also at greater risk for maltreatment (Boyce, Behl, Moretensen, & Akers, 1991; Committee on Child Abuse and Neglect and Committee on Children With Disabilities, 2001; Streeck-Fischer & van der Kolk, 2000; Sullivan & Knutson, 2000).

Family factors such as poor parenting skills and the use of harsh discipline may also put a child at risk for maltreatment (DePanfilis, 1998; Straus, 2000). The majority of abuse that occurs to children with disabilities occurs in their homes, so careful family assessment is particularly important.

Societal Contributions to Risk

A number of systems contributions to increased risk for maltreatment of children with disabilities need to be considered when working with an abused child or adult survivor of abuse. Societal attitudes that view children and people with disabilities as deviant, or popular and news media that refuse to normalize the experiences of individuals with disabilities, contribute to the vulnerability of individuals with disabilities (Davis, 2001). Medical and mental health systems can increase children's vulnerability to maltreatment by not providing adequate care to a child with disabilities or by encouraging disengagement of family members from a child, such as a newborn with serious disabilities (Mitchell & Buchele-Ash, 2000).

Education systems also can increase the risk for maltreatment when the education provided is inadequate for preparing a child with disabilities for adult life, or for his or her day-to-day life as a child or teen, or when family members are excluded as team members (Weinberg, 1997). Systems that encourage programs of isolation or enforce zero-tolerance programs on children who, because of their disability, may not adequately manage normative social behaviors (Huchet, 2001), may also increase the risk for abuse.

Recent studies show that teachers' perceptions of the severity of the disability influence the attitudes they hold toward their included students with disabilities: Children with hidden disabilities, such as learning disabilities, are more likely to engender intolerance in teachers than are children with more obvious disabilities, such as orthopedic disabilities or autism (Cook, 2001).

Social service systems that provide services to children with disabilities are sometimes separate from child protective systems and may differ in their eligibility requirements and age cutoffs. This puts children with disabilities at risk for falling through the cracks and not receiving the care they need. Depending on the severity of the disability, out-of-home options may not be available for a maltreated child with disabilities. Policymakers increase the vulnerability of children with disabilities when they do not pass laws at the federal and state levels and when they cut social service budgets that support the protection of children with disabilities (Mitchell & Buchele-Ash, 2000; Pear & Toner, 2002).

REPORTING AND ASSESSMENT ISSUES

Barriers to Disclosure and Reporting

Many factors influence whether a report of maltreatment is made to the appropriate authorities when a child with disabilities is abused or neglected. Individuals who have the potential to report maltreatment often lack sufficient training to identify the signs and symptoms of abuse and neglect, especially when the child has a disability (Mitchell & Buchele-Ash, 2000). Potential reporters may believe that reporting will lead to further harm, may lack confidence in the protective service system, or may fear that it will harm their relationship with the family (Mitchell & Buchele-Ash, 2000).

However, children with disabilities may face some unique barriers to disclosure. Depending on the type of disability, children with disabilities may not be able to disclose their abuse because of communication difficulties (Albin, 1992; McCreary & Thompson, 1999; Sullivan & Knutson, 1998). Some children with disabilities may not be able to discriminate the occurrence of a crime if it was not physically painful. They may lack the skills or physical capacities to challenge, escape, or report it (Clees & Gast, 1994). Children with disabilities may fear disclosing the abuse if they are dependent on the perpetrator for direct care and support services.

Children with disabilities, especially those who live in institutions, may be more isolated than children without disabilities. Gaining access to safe, trustworthy adults may be more difficult for them (Committee on Child Abuse and Neglect and Committee on Children With Disabilities, 2001). Finally, children with disabilities, especially developmental disabilities, may not be believed even if they can recount their experiences of abuse (Sobsey & Mansell, 1990; Tharinger, Horton, & Millea, 1990).

Assessment

The heterogeneity of children with disabilities and their families calls for a broad and comprehensive approach to assessment and evaluation (Ammerman, 1997). No two children or families are alike when it comes to problems, symptoms, or skill deficits. The evaluation of children with disabilities demands many of the same assessment procedures and tools that a clinician would use when treating a child without disabilities. Carefully evaluating the specifics of the abuse situation; assessing the family environment and parent–child relationship; and then examining other social units that interact with the family, including school, work, other caregivers, and friends, is crucial for a comprehensive evaluation (Clees & Gast, 1994).

TREATMENT ISSUES

There is scant research on how to respond to children with disabilities who have been maltreated (Orelove, Hollahan, & Myles, 2000). Gaps in services are widespread, and counseling services are often inaccessible, unavailable, or not appropriately modified for the individual child (Mansell et. al., 1998). Disabled children may not be offered services that are as extensive or intensive as services offered to children without disabilities (Albin, 1992; Hollins & Sinason, 2000). Inpatient adolescent units are sometimes not equipped to work with a child with a developmental delay who may need more one-on-one attention than the other patients.

Programs for children with disabilities that target the treatment and prevention of abuse and neglect are beginning to appear and should be based on research-derived risk factors and empirical evaluation (Clees & Gast, 1994; Orelove et al., 2000; Sullivan & Cork, 1998). There is, however, a sizable gap between clinical practice and empirical outcome studies that demonstrate their effectiveness with children who have disabilities (Shirk & Eltz, 1998). This is also true for the efficacy of parent education for caregivers who abuse their children (Reppucci, Britner, & Woolard, 1997).

Prevention efforts that target the different adults in various micro-systems of the individual child's life are the goal of choice for treatment (Sullivan & Cork, 1998). Collaboration across all professions—including teachers, physicians, nurses, mental health practitioners, police, prosecutors and judges, advocates, and child protective workers—is viewed as an essential focus of ecological treatment (Orelove et al., 2000). Prevention efforts geared primarily toward training professionals to teach children how to protect themselves are not recommended for children with disabilities (Sullivan & Cork, 1998). The responsibility for protection should not be placed on the child; efforts should be addressed to the total ecological system of the child (Sullivan & Cork, 1998).

For clinicians, it is important to have information and training on types of disabilities, developmental stages and delays, maltreatment vulnerabilities, methods of working with individuals with disabilities, and resources (Batshaw, 1997; Sullivan & Cork, 1998). Requesting or seeking out continuing education in this area is important (Orelove et al., 2000). Every state has an office on mental retardation or developmental disabilities that can provide names of agencies and institutions that provide training and have information. Treatment and prevention of the victimization of children with disabilities also have to include providing resources and education to parents, educators, legal professionals, and social service caseworkers.

Impact of Abuse

The impact of abuse on children with disabilities is thought to be not all that different from that for children without disabilities (Mansell et al., 1998). However, it should be noted that there is a paucity of literature on the actual health outcomes or health problems for children with disabilities who have been abused, so the empirical basis for this assumption is unsubstantiated. Chronic childhood exposure to family violence and trauma interferes with the capacity for normal development and inflicts a host of devastating symptoms on children. The effects of family violence and child abuse can also cause neurological sequelae and injury to the brain and spinal cord in young children, and under certain circumstances it can cause nonorganic failure to thrive, pseudoseizures, and left-hemisphere deficits (Cahill, Kaminer, & Johnson, 1999). In the area of school performance, children who have been maltreated may experience language delays and adverse academic outcomes, such as poorer grades, more suspensions, and more grade repetitions (Kendall-Tackett & Eckenrode, 1996). Child maltreatment can also cause a plethora of devastating negative mental health outcomes and psychological symptoms, including anxious attachments, posttraumatic stress disorder, and depression. There may also be problems with oppositional behavior; emotional self-regulation; and regulation of affect, impulse control, and aggression toward self and others (Mullen, Martin, Anderson, Romans, & Herbison, 1996; Streeck-Fischer & van der Kolk, 2000).

As with children who do not have disabilities, children with disabilities who have been maltreated may develop self-harming behaviors. It is unfortunate that in the past these behaviors have been attributed to the disability and have rarely been viewed as a symptom of possible abuse, as they are in children without disabilities (Downie, 2001; Mansell et al., 1998). Clinicians need to be cognizant that the same signs and symptoms in nondisabled children may appear in children with disabilities.

Some abuse issues, however, appear to be compounded for children with disabilities by factors related to the disability, particularly when the disability is a developmental one. The experience of social isolation and dependency on others, particularly family members, can increase the child's anxiety, anger, and fear of retaliation and abandonment (Mansell et al., 1998). Inadequate knowledge of and comfort with sexuality and normative social behavior, and the ability to understand what are safe and unsafe environments, may complicate the child's understanding of his or her abuse (Clees & Gast, 1994; Mansell et al., 1998).

Trauma can magnify speech and communication problems in individuals with developmental disabilities. These children may be more confused and have a greater difficulty understanding their abuse and communicating about it (Mansell et al., 1998). Depending on the type of disability, the child with disabilities may be more susceptible to psychological problems and may experience the trauma as more devastating than a child without a disability (Mansell et al., 1998).

Goals of Treatment

The goals of treatment for children with disabilities who have been maltreated are to alleviate guilt; repair trust; overcome depression, posttraumatic stress disorder, and self-harming behaviors; improve self-esteem; and, for older children and youth, teach self-protective strategies (Mansell et al., 1998). In addition, stopping the abuse and seeing to it that all the players in the child's life are educated about his or her disability requires a high level of collaboration and coordination.

All treatment occurs in the context of a therapeutic relationship and the development of a therapeutic alliance. The development of a treatment alliance is a challenging task with children who have been abused at the hands of caregivers, and maltreated children with disabilities are no exception. It may, however, require a greater commitment from the clinician. Clinicians need to believe that children with disabilities who have been maltreated deserve and need the same care, sustenance, and specialized interventions that their nondisabled peers receive.

CONCLUSION

Child clinicians need to raise their awareness regarding the maltreatment of children with disabilities, identify gaps in the services to these children, and develop and promote service delivery models that meet these children's special needs. Clinicians need to encourage and support research on the needs of children with disabilities to make their practices evidence based. Finally, clinicians need to educate themselves, question their own assumptions, and apply ecological perspectives to understand the multiplicative impacts and vulnerabilities of children with disabilities and the adults they become.

REFERENCES

Albin, J. (1992). Sexual abuse in young children with developmental disabilities: Assessment and treatment issues. *Journal of Developmental Disabilities, 1,* 29–40.

Ammerman, R. T. (1997). Physical abuse and childhood disability: Risk factors and treatment factors. *Journal of Aggression, Maltreatment and Trauma, 1,* 207–225.

Batshaw, M. (Ed.). (1997). *Children with disabilities* (4th ed.). Baltimore: Brookes Publishing.

Belsky, J. (1993). Etiology of child maltreatment: A developmental–ecological analysis. *Psychological Bulletin, 14,* 413–434.

Boyce, C., Behl, D., Moretensen, L., & Akers, J. (1991). Child characteristics, family demographics and family processes: Their effects on the stress experienced by families of children with disabilities. *Counseling Psychology Quarterly, 4,* 273–288.

Cahill, L. T., Kaminer, R. K., & Johnson, P. G. (1999). Developmental, cognitive, and behavioral sequelae of child abuse. *Child and Adolescent Psychiatric Clinics of North America, 8,* 827–842.

Clees, T., & Gast, D. (1994). Social safety skills instruction for individuals with disabilities: A sequential model. *Education and Treatment of Children, 1,* 163–184.

Coleman, A. (1997). Disability. *Youth Studies Australia, 16*(2), 6–8.

Committee on Child Abuse and Neglect and Committee on Children With Disabilities. (2001). Assessment of maltreatment of children with disabilities. *American Academy of Pediatrics, 108,* 508–512.

Cook, B. G. (2001). A comparison of teachers' attitudes toward their included students with mild and severe disabilities. *Journal of Special Education, 34,* 203–214.

Cook, B. G., & Semmel, M. (1999). Peer acceptance of included students with disabilities as a function of severity of disability and classroom composition. *Journal of Special Education, 33*(10), 50–62.

Davis, L. J. (2001). J'accuse!: Cultural imperialism—Ableist style. *Social Alternatives, 18*(1), 36–41.

De Panfilis, D. (1998). Intervening with families when children are neglected. In H. Dubowitz (Ed.), *Neglected children: Research, practice and policy* (pp. 211–236). Thousand Oaks, CA: Sage.

Downie, S. (2001). Falling through the gap: Women with mild learning disabilities and self-harm. *Feminist Review, 68,* 177–181.

Embry, R. A. (2001, July). *Examination of risk factors for maltreatment of deaf children: Findings from a national survey.* Paper presented at the 7th International Family Violence Research conference, Portsmouth, NH.

Finkelhor, D., Mitchell, K., & Wolak, J. (2000). *Online victimization: A report on the nation's youth.* Washington, DC: U.S. Department of Justice.

Grauerholz, L. (2000). An ecological approach to understanding sexual revictimization: Linking personal, interpersonal, and socio-cultural factors and processes. *Child Maltreatment, 5,* 5–17.

Hollins, S., & Sinason, V. (2000). Psychotherapy, learning disabilities and trauma: New perspectives. *British Journal of Psychiatry, 176,* 32–36.

Huchet, C. G. (2001, Winter). Zero tolerance = zero thinking = zero sense: A school policy that places our kids at risk. *The Source,* pp. 1–3.

Kendall-Tackett, K. A., & Eckenrode, J. (1996). The effects of neglect on academic achievement and disciplinary problems: A developmental perspective. *Child Abuse and Neglect, 20*, 161–170.

Little, L. (2002). Middle-class mothers' perceptions of peer and sibling victimization among children with Asperger's Syndrome and nonverbal learning disorders. *Issues in Comprehensive Pediatric Nursing, 25*, 43–57.

Llewellyn, A. (1995). The abuse of children with physical disabilities in mainstream schooling. *Developmental Medicine and Child Neurology, 37*, 740–743.

Llewellyn, A., & Hogan, K. (2000). The use and abuse models of disability. *Disability and Society, 15*, 157–165.

Mansell, S., Sobsey, D., & Moskal, R. (1998). Clinical findings among sexually abused children with and without developmental disabilities. *Mental Retardation, 36*, 12–22.

McCreary, B. D., & Thompson, J. (1999). Psychiatric aspects of sexual abuse involving persons with developmental disabilities. *Canadian Journal of Psychiatry, 44*, 350–355.

Mitchell, L., & Buchele-Ash, A. (2000). Abuse and neglect of individuals with disabilities: Building protective supports through public policy. *Journal of Disability Policy Studies, 10*, 225–243.

Morrison, G., Furlong, M., & Smith, G. (1994). Factors associated with the experience of school violence among general education, leadership class, opportunity class, and special day class pupils. *Education and Treatment of Children, 17*, 356–369.

Mullen, P. E., Martin, J. L., Anderson, J. C., Romans, S. E., & Herbison, G. P. (1996). The long-term impact of the physical, emotional, and sexual abuse of children: A community study. *Child Abuse and Neglect, 20*, 7–21.

National Center on Child Abuse and Neglect. (1993). *A report on the maltreatment of children with disabilities* (DHHS Contract No. 105-89-1630). Washington, DC: Author.

National Clearinghouse on Child Abuse and Neglect Information. (2001). *The risk and prevention of maltreatment of children with disabilities.* Retrieved June 23, 2003, from http://www.calib.com/nccanch/pubs/prevenres/focus.cfm

Orelove, F. P., Hollahan, D. J., & Myles, K. T. (2000). Maltreatment of children with disabilities: Training needs for a collaborative response. *Child Abuse and Neglect, 24*, 185–194.

Pear, R., & Toner, R. (2002, January 14). Grim choices face states in making cuts in Medicaid. *The New York Times*, pp. A1, A13.

Reppucci, N. D., Britner, P. A., & Woolard, J. A (1997). *Preventing child abuse and neglect through parent education.* Baltimore: Brookes Publishing.

Rodriguez, C. M., & Murphy, L. (1997). Parenting stress and abuse potential in mothers of children with developmental disabilities. *Child Maltreatment, 2*, 245–252.

Santich, M., & Kavanagh, D. (1997). Social adaptation of children with mild intellectual disability: Effects of partial integration within primary school classes. *Australian Psychologist, 32,* 126–130.

Shirk, S., & Eltz, M. (1998). Multiple victimization in the process and outcome of child psychotherapy. In B. B. Rossman & M. Rosenburg (Eds.), *Multiple victimizations of children: Conceptual, developmental, research and treatment issues* (pp. 233–253). Binghamton, NY: Haworth.

Sobsey, D., & Mansell, S. (1990). The prevention of sexual abuse of people with developmental disabilities. *Developmental Disabilities Bulletin, 18*(2), 51–66.

Sobsey, R., Randall, W., & Parrila, R. K. (1997). Gender differences in abused children with and without disabilities. *Child Abuse and Neglect, 21,* 707–720.

Straus, M. A. (2000). *Beating the devil out of them: Corporal punishment in American families* (2nd ed.). Boston: Lexington Books.

Streeck-Fischer, A., & van der Kolk, B. (2000). Down will come baby, cradle and all: Diagnostic and therapeutic implications of chronic trauma on child development. *Australian and New Zealand Journal of Psychiatry, 34,* 903–918.

Sullivan, P., & Cork, P. (1998). Maltreatment prevention programs for children with disabilities: An evaluation model. *Developmental Disabilities Bulletin, 26*(1), 59–70.

Sullivan, P., & Knutson, J. (1998). The association between child maltreatment and disabilities in a hospital-based epidemiological study. *Child Abuse and Neglect, 22,* 271–288.

Sullivan, P. M., & Knutson, J. F. (2000). Maltreatment and disabilities: A population-based epidemiological study. *Child Abuse and Neglect, 24,* 1257–1273.

Tharinger, D., Horton, C. B., & Millea, S. (1990). Sexual abuse and exploitation of children and adults with mental retardation and other handicaps. *Child Abuse and Neglect, 14,* 301–312.

Thompson, D., Whitney, I., & Smith, P. (1994). Bullying of children with special needs in mainstream schools. *Support for Learning, 9,* 103–106.

U.S. Department of Health and Human Services. (1997). *Trends in the well-being of America's children and youth.* Washington, DC: Author.

Weinberg, L. (1997). Problems in educating abused and neglected children with disabilities. *Child Abuse and Neglect, 21,* 889–905.

Westat Inc. (1993). *A report on the maltreatment of children with disabilities.* Washington, DC: National Center on Child Abuse and Neglect.

7

ELDER ABUSE: CLINICAL ASSESSMENT AND OBLIGATION TO REPORT

Elder abuse is a common but underreported type of family violence; one that is intimately linked with health. Elder abuse and neglect often take place in the context of illness and caretaking issues. It can cause or exacerbate medical conditions, and it often presents in health care settings. This chapter explores the phenomenon of domestic elder abuse in the United States and provides an overview of elder abuse protection laws. Victims and perpetrators are profiled using case examples and flow charts to assist health care providers in detecting suspected abuse. The important role of health care professionals in conducting elder abuse screening assessments and their obligation to report suspicion of elder abuse are presented.

Of all the forms of family violence, elder abuse has received the least attention in the family violence and health care literature. Yet estimates of incidents of elder abuse range from 700,000 to 2 million annually (Jordan, 2001), with most of the abuse perpetrated by family members. Only 16% of these cases are reported to the proper agency (National Elder Abuse Incidence Study [NEAIS], 1998). Self-neglecting older people, who often severely compromise their own health by not attending to their physical needs or home environment, numbered about 101,000 in 1996 (NEAIS, 1998).

Elder abuse exists in all socioeconomic classes and affects both men and women, although women are abused in greater numbers. It is expected that cases of elder abuse will continue to rise as the U.S. population ages. Some factors contributing to the expected increase are decreased birth rates, increased longevity, improved medical care, more women who are in the workforce and unavailable for full- and part-time caregiving of relatives, acceptance of divorce and remarriage among all age groups, ill-preparedness among traditional family care providers (Kosberg & Garcia, 1995b), a lack of federal and state support for aged programs, and a sense of complacency among the public and professionals regarding issues of elder abuse.

Psychologists and other mental health professionals are in an ideal position to assist older people trapped in abusive situations. Often, the illnesses and symptoms (e.g., dementia, depression, aggression due to stroke or brain injury, or behavioral problems) that promote older people or their caregivers to seek out mental health professionals are primary indicators of potential elder abuse. For example, Dyer, Pavlik, Murphy, and Hyman (2000) found that neglected or abused older people have much higher rates of depression and dementia. Mental health professionals are also instrumental in assisting with competency evaluations, which have an important role in the elder abuse field. An incompetent older person is more susceptible to abuse and can be directed to accept services by elder abuse practitioners. A competent older person will remain in charge of his or her living situation should allegations of abuse be confirmed. Most mental health practitioners already have a knowledge base from which to assess elder abuse because they are trained assessors for child and partner abuse. Many of the same risk factors apply to elder abuse by family members. Consequently, mental health professionals are in strategic positions to assess and to report suspected cases of elder abuse.

In this chapter I briefly outline the various forms of familial elder abuse, elder abuse reporting laws and reporting obligations for professionals, and basic assessment strategies. I focus on domestic (noninstitutional) abuse of elderly individuals, with a focus on abuse involving a perpetrator versus self-neglecting older people. I do not address developmental or disabled adults younger than age 60, a population included in many adult and elder abuse reporting laws. Because elder abuse is underreported by health care and mental health professionals, the purpose of this chapter is to highlight the main role of the health care professions in the detection and reporting of elder abuse and the provision of supportive services to reduce and eliminate abuse in substantiated cases. The chapter concludes with a list of resources for helping professionals further their knowledge on this topic.

CLASSIFICATION OF ELDER ABUSE

Abuse of elderly people occurs in several ways, and often the types of abuse overlap with one another. Self-neglect—a competent older person's lack of attention to his or her health and physical well-being needs—constitutes the largest category of elder abuse and is the only form of abuse that does not involve a perpetrator. The other classifications of elder abuse include passive and active neglect (including abandonment); psychological, physical, and sexual abuse; and financial exploitation (NEAIS, 1998). Of all of the classifications, there is the most agreement around what constitutes physical abuse, whereas sexual abuse of elderly people is the least studied of the classifications (Loue, 2001). All classifications of abuse are considered to be reportable to authorized state agencies and are described in Exhibit 7.1. Because of space limitations, this chapter will not focus on forms of elder neglect, although that too is a significant health care problem.

ELDER ABUSE AS A HEALTH ISSUE

Unlike domestic violence, few studies look at elder abuse as a health issue. However, the World Health Organization cites elder abuse, along with other forms of violence, as an international health care issue consisting of many complex factors (Krug, Mercy, Dahlberg, & Zwl, 2002). Also, the Wisconsin Department of Health and Social Services found in 1998 that 10% of all reported cases involved a life-threatening situation, and 12 deaths were recorded in a single year (Welfel, Danzinger, & Santoro, 2000). Wolf (1997, cited in Welfel et al., 2000) clearly documented that abuse contributes to common forms of psychological dysfunction, including depression, post-traumatic stress, learned helplessness, and alienation. In addition, elderly people who are abused begin to isolate themselves because of feelings of fear, shame, and guilt (Welfel et al., 2000), or their perpetrator isolates them to gain greater control over them. This isolation further confounds detection of and intervention in elder abuse cases.

Because elder abuse is a complex health care phenomenon, and both public and professional education has lagged behind that of other forms of intrafamily violence, health care costs resulting from elder abuse have not been tracked. However, the domestic violence literature is rich with research focused on the health consequences of domestic abuse involving younger victims. The direct cost of treating victims of domestic violence for health and mental health issues is approximately $1.8 billion each year (Miller, Cohen & Wierseman, 1995, as cited in Gerlock, 1999). It may be reasonable to assume that many issues of elder health care could be a result of perpetrator acts of abuse. Some of these health effects include dehydration, inappropriate

EXHIBIT 7.1
Classification of Elder Abuse

Self-Neglect
> An older person's willful or unintentional self-care, a lack of attention to the environment, resulting in unhealthy and unsafe conditions

Passive-Unintentional Caregiver Neglect
> A primary caregiver's lack of attention to the basic daily care, social, recreational, and health needs of an older person that compromises the overall well-being of an older person and his or her quality of life; a lack of attention to the older person's physical surroundings, resulting in unhealthy and unsafe conditions

Active-Intentional Caregiver Neglect
> A primary caregiver's willful intention to withhold or refuse the basic daily care or social, recreational, and health needs of an older person that compromises the overall well-being of an older person and his or her quality of life; a lack of attention to the older person's physical surroundings, resulting in unhealthy and unsafe conditions

Psychological Abuse
> A perpetrator's verbal aggression or emotional abuse (e.g., abusive language, threats) of an older person that induces fear, intimidation, lower self-esteem, and reduced functioning

Physical Abuse
> A perpetrator's action (restraining, slapping, shoving, burning, biting, etc.) toward an older person that produces pain or injury

Sexual Abuse
> A perpetrator's infliction of unwanted intimate behavior on an older person, including sexual talk; the showing of pictures or films that are sexual in nature; committing sexual acts in the presence of the elder; and touching the older person physically in any intimate manner, including sexual intercourse

Financial Exploitation
> A perpetrator's misuse or illegal use of an elder's money and assets, including savings, investments, property, and belongings, for the perpetrator's self-gain or the gain of others

medication intake, malnutrition and poor nutrition, compromised skin conditions, lacerations, falls, fractures, substance abuse, urinary tract infection, lacerations around the genitals, sexually transmitted disease, late onset of AIDS, or bruising. There may also be complications of health due to poor environment or extreme isolation, and this can contribute to anxiety and depression. Risk factors for abuse are all seen in home health care, mental health clinics, emergency departments, and acute settings, as well as in long-term institutional care.

It is therefore vital for good health care of older people that physicians, psychologists, nurses, medical social workers, counselors, and other health professionals know how to screen for suspected abuse and make appropriate referrals to designated state agencies.

ELDER ABUSE AND NEGLECT-REPORTING LAWS

Although elder abuse reporting laws exist in every state, professionals tend to hesitate in reporting their suspicions of elder abuse. Several reasons have been attributed to this lack of reporting. Professionals may be ignorant of the elder abuse reporting law in their state (Ehrlich & Anetzberger, 1991), or they may lack the necessary knowledge and training to assess for elder abuse. Agencies and organizations who provide services to elderly people (e.g., mental health clinics) may lack policies and procedures for reporting elder abuse (Ehrlich & Anetzberger, 1991), although such policies may exist for child abuse reporting. Furthermore, state laws lack universal standards and definitions of abuse and neglect, and the agency to which one should report suspected elder abuse varies from state to state (Ehrlich & Anetzberger, 1991). This lack of consistency can make it difficult for professionals providing services to clients, especially if their practice spans several different states. Still, these inconsistencies do not relieve professionals from their obligation to assess for elder abuse and report their suspicions of abuse. Last, there is a pervasive ageism in U.S. society that affects the attitudes of professionals about treating older clients and policies initiated for servicing older clients in the health and mental health care systems (Schneewind, 1994; Wolf, 1996).

Duty to Report

In general, elder abuse laws are designed to protect both competent and incompetent older individuals as long as the elderly victim is "vulnerable" in some way. The term *vulnerable* usually has a vague description in the law but tends to imply that the elderly person is frail; dependent on a caregiver for physical care, management of finances, or in-home services; is suffering from an illness; is developmentally challenged, mildly confused, or clearly demented; or a combination of any of these. Some elder abuse experts argue that a history of domestic violence may also make an elderly person vulnerable to abuse in old age (Bergeron, 2001; Brandl & Raymond, 1997; Harris, 1996). Not every state law mandates that suspicions of elder abuse be reported. Some states instead encourage reporting but consider it a voluntary action at the discretion of the professional (for a discussion on state laws, see Welfel et al., 2000). Nevertheless, all laws include the duty of professionals, particularly those in counseling fields, to report if either they suspect abuse or they become knowledgeable through a credible source that abuse may be occurring.

The laws protect reporters of elder abuse from civil lawsuit if there is no malicious intent and preserve the reporters' confidentiality. However, when professionals report abuse, it may be more appropriate for them to inform the elderly person as part of the therapeutic intervention rather than withhold that information. If the state law mandates reporting, professionals should state that they are making a report because of their legal obligation to do so, just as in child abuse cases. If the state law permits voluntary reporting, professionals may cite their ethical obligation to report clients at risk. In both situations, concern for the client's safety should be cited as a paramount reason for reporting. Last, professionals are not expected to verify abuse but need only to present their suspicions of abuse with the evidence and information they have available. It is the duty of the elder abuse practitioner to verify abuse through the authorized state investigative process.

Currently, elder abuse laws are social service based, and elder abuse protective (EAP) practitioners usually approach each reported case as an investigator and problem-solver. These practitioners are well acquainted with area resources and programs for troubled older people and their families. Many state laws also provide authority to EAP practitioners to obtain bank records and medical reports during the investigative process. All laws are rooted in the principle of the competent elderly person's right to self-determine the intervention process, even if abuse is substantiated. Therefore, a report of suspected elder abuse does not remove an older person from his or her home. Neither does it force undesirable choices on the elderly person (Bergeron, 2000). Reports may also be made many times on one client. Hence, if an older person is suspected of being abused, and a report is made, it does not preclude another report in the future if abuse is still suspected. Often, the filing of multiple reports allows EAP practitioners a rapport-building process so that over time victims who hesitated in accepting services will begin to do so.

Reporting Guidelines

Welfel et al. (2000) delineated five guidelines for practitioners in reporting their suspicions of elder abuse. First, practitioners must accept that elder abuse happens frequently enough that every elderly client should be screened for possible abuse. Second, practitioners should ask nonconfrontational or nonaccusatory questions when they screen for abuse. Welfel et al. suggested a simple question such as "Do you feel safe in your home?" An attitude of helping, versus a confrontational or inquisitional style, should prevail in the assessment process. Third, practitioners need to become aware of risk factors indicating abuse. Fourth, family members should be interviewed separately; and fifth, practitioners must become knowledgeable about services for older people and make appropriate referrals for the elderly person and his or her caregiver.

ASSESSMENT: IDENTIFYING RISK FACTORS

Assessment of abuse can be extremely complex. Practitioners base their assessments on the visual observation of the elderly client and the relative or caregiver providing support to the client. Knowledge of family systems, personality theory, interviewing techniques, and competency evaluations are part of assessing for elder abuse. These skills are often already a part of the mental health practitioner's repertoire. Understanding the normal aging process is equally important so that one can distinguish factors related to disease versus abuse. For example, a statement of "My daughter is taking all my money" may be an actual fact, or it may reflect paranoia caused by dementia.

Elder abuse can present in a number of ways. Risk factors, if viewed separately, may not be viewed as a cause for great concern, but when taken together they paint a portrait of an older person in need of intervention. Health care professionals have the primary duty to detect, report, and provide ongoing supportive services. The task of substantiating abuse or neglect resides within the designated state agency of elder protection. (For a concise discussion of various assessment tools and referral protocol, see Anetzberger, 2001.

Older victims may present with depression, anxiety, low self-worth, or substance abuse (including abuse of prescription medications). They may report a long history of family dysfunction or have lived with their caretaker for more than 10 years. They may be hesitant to express opinions, especially in front of the perpetrator. They may report being restricted within the home, having no access to certain rooms, food, the telephone, or they may report being left out of family gatherings.

Some physical signs of ongoing abuse include injuries such as bruises around the wrist, leg, or waist (possibly indicating the use of restraints); bruises around the neck or throat; bruises in "hidden" areas such as the scalp, thighs, vaginal area, or the soles of the feet; bite marks; or circular burns. Physical signs of active or passive neglect include long, curling toenails; malnutrition; dehydration; and lack of functional aids such as hearing aids, glasses, false teeth, or medicines (Baron & Welty, 1996; Dyer et al., 2000; Fulmer, 1991; Kallman, 1987; Kosberg & Garcia, 1995a; Penhale, 1999; Peterson & Paris, 1995; Schiamberg & Gans, 2000; Shock, 2000; Sijuwade, 1995; Welfel et al., 2000; Wolf, 1996).

FAMILY MEMBERS AS ABUSERS AND VICTIMS

Older people living in the community are subject to abuse primarily by family members. Adult children, followed by spouses, represent the largest group of perpetrators of elder abuse (NEAIS, 1998). This is not surprising since most of the supportive care received by community dwelling elders is from family members. In order for health care providers to make sound assessments of elder abuse, it is critical that they understand some of the causal theoretical models as to why some family members are abusive to older relatives, how the relationship of adult, child, or spouse to the alleged elder victim complicates the assessment process, and the various risk factors that make an older person susceptible to being abused.

Theoretical Models for Abuse of Older People

Theories of caregiver stress and burden-of-care have been the primary models used to explain elder abuse at the hands of family members. The caregiver stress model asserts that abuse occurs because of stressors in the caregiver's life, causing a lashing out by the caregiver at the care receiver. Although researchers now believe that this theory of causation is representative of a small percentage of those family members who abuse and that this model has been oversimplified (Anetzberger, 2000), it is critical that health care providers are capable of assessing the burden-of-care felt by family members. If abuse is due to the caregiver being over-burdened, a primary function of the health care provider is not just assessing for abuse, but also imparting knowledge of community services available to assist in the older person's care, and in educating caregivers about abuse and neglect.

Overwhelmed or overburdened caregivers are often forthcoming in telling about their living situation. Well-meaning caregivers usually are respectful of (although maybe frustrated with) the older person, concerned for his or her welfare versus their own welfare, and want to do a good job. Consequently, they are usually apologetic or guilt ridden about any injury to the older person that they may have caused. Many are open to receiving help from the outside, and those who are not initially receptive may be challenged to accept assistance (Lechner, 1993). However, well-intended caregivers abusing an older person because of burden and stress are not to be excused from their actions. Professionals in the field have an obligation not to make excuses for perpetrators of elder abuse, because doing so justifies and inadvertently supports their abusive actions (Brandl & Raymond, 1997).

Current research findings, however, suggest that caregiver stress is an inadequate explanation for all elder abuse (Anetzberger, 2000; Bergeron, 2001; Brandl & Raymond, 1997; Dunlop, Rothman, Condon, Hebert, & Martinez, 2000; Reis & Nahmiash, 1997). Such theories have inadvertently impeded the understanding and securitization of suspected elder abuse victims receiving health care. Consequently, professionals must move beyond the parochial constraints of the caregiver-stress model when confronted with suspicions that an older person may not be receiving adequate care to assess the motivation and intention of the caregiver (Anetzberger, 2000). Viewing suspected elderly victims living with family members as possible victims of domestic violence is useful, because instead of looking at the burden of care, the focus is on the development of the relationship and assessment of family interactions and levels of power (Seaver, 1996). As in other phenomena of domestic violence, it is the unequal use of power that evolves over time and serves the needs of perpetrators that promotes some of the more serious cases of familial elder abuse.

Abuse by Adult Children

Older people being abused by their adult children may be reluctant to seek help for a variety of reasons, but paramount among these is a desire to still provide for one's children. This is especially true if the child has issues of substance abuse, need for housing, or has developmental or mental health issues. Many people with mental disabilities were deinstitutionalized in the 1960s and returned to live with their families of origin. Deinstitutionalized people and their caretakers are now 30 or more years older and may be in compromising situations because of their advancing age, frailties of health, household and money management issues, and role reversal of caretaking due to age.

Abuse by Spouses

Older people being abused by spouses may be of two types: (a) early-onset abuse, in which there is a long-term history of domestic violence within the marriage, and (b) late-onset spousal abuse, in which there is recent spousal aggression. Sometimes late-onset abuse is due to pathology that changes the spouse's behavior (e.g., aggression due to dementia), or it is linked to late onset of alcoholism, or it may be a result of a new relationship resulting in marriage or cohabitation. Some other risk factors include a previously abusive spouse now frail and dependent for care combined with the notion of "payback" by the once-victimized spouse-turned-caregiver. Substance abuse by the spousal perpetrator, high levels of marital conflict or verbal aggression, depression, or a significant life change are also risk factors for spousal abuse (Dunlop et al., 2000; Harris, 1996; Vinton, 1992). The abused older person may hesitate to seek help so as not to burden the adult children with either his or her physical care or with the care of the impaired (e.g., by substance abuse or mental illness) spousal perpetrator. These concerns increase if the perpetrator abused the children when they were young.

Risk Factors for Abuse

Dependency increases the risk for elder abuse victims. Older individuals unable to care for their own activities of daily living, or who experience psychological problems (e.g., some level of dementia, or depression) are more likely to be abused. The age of the older person has been found to be a significant risk factor, with those 75 years and older more likely to be at risk (Cyphers, 1999). The older person's attitude toward receiving care is an important factor in risk for abuse. Older individuals who are neurotic or disagreeable (Reis & Nahmiash, 1997), ungrateful, or self-determining of their own neglectful situations are more likely to suffer abuse and neglect. Older people who are fearful or afraid of upsetting their care providers, thereby being accepting and complying even when being victimized, or who accept responsibility for their relatives' well-being, will more likely be victims of abuse (Schiamberg & Gans, 2000).

There are also risk factors associated with the caregivers beyond burden of care. Evaluating for dependency of the caregiver on the older person, substance abuse, financial difficulties, depression, and personality disorders is helpful in making a distinction from burden of care. Ascertaining whether people in the household lead an unhealthy lifestyle or have developmental, psychological, or physical impairments should also be noted as risk factors (Schiamberg & Gans, 2000). In addition to evaluating the older person's risk for abuse, one must determine the older person's assessment of his or her caregiver (Peterson & Paris, 1995). Inquiries should focus on the older person's feelings of responsibility for the welfare of the relative or caregiver and issues of violence involving the relative or caregiver.

Personality traits may also be an indicator of possible risk factors to the older person (Ramsey-Klawsnik, 2000; Reis & Nahmiash, 1997). Of particular note is the personality factor of neuroticism and agreeableness of the victim (Reis & Nahmiash, 1997) and the personality traits of narcissism and sadism of the perpetrator (Ramsey-Klawsnik, 2000).

In this next section, I provide some case examples that illustrate the interplay between victim and perpetrator risk factors.

CASE EXAMPLES

Stephen and Al

Stephen, aged 75, was living with his son Al, who was 58 years old and unemployed. Stephen entered the emergency room with a possible hip fracture and shoulder dislocation after a fall. Al accompanied him to the emergency room and asked to be present for any interviews because his

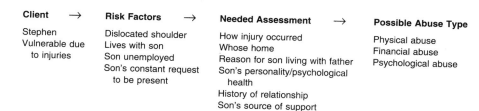

Client	→	Risk Factors	→	Needed Assessment	→	Possible Abuse Type
Stephen Vulnerable due to injuries		Dislocated shoulder Lives with son Son unemployed Son's constant request to be present		How injury occurred Whose home Reason for son living with father Son's personality/psychological health History of relationship Son's source of support		Physical abuse Financial abuse Psychological abuse

Figure 7.1. A case of possible physical abuse.

father was disoriented. He answered most of the questions asked of his father. Although the son appeared to be somewhat controlling, he was also engaging with the staff and appeared concerned about his father's welfare. The case is illustrated in Figure 7.1.

Because family members perpetrate most elder abuse in domestic settings, it is important to assess the relationship the elderly individual has with family members. Excluding neglect, men commit more abuse of older people by a ratio of 3:2 (Cyphers, 1999; NEAIS, 1998). Most perpetrators typically are younger than their victims, although in cases of spousal abuse age may not be a factor (Cyphers, 1999).

In this case, Stephen represents a possible case of physical abuse. Because Stephen's son Al is unemployed and may be dependent on him for support, this case may also represent financial exploitation, which is often coupled with psychological abuse. Al's interaction with the health care professionals may be interpreted as concern for his father's welfare, or he may be controlling his father's interactions to avoid detection of abuse.

In addition to the perpetrator's relationship to the victim, there are other factors useful in assessing for possible abuse. Admission or intake forms often ask whether older people are living alone and with whom they live; however, they do not ask who owns the home. This is important information, because it may indicate issues of control. For example, in the above case, it may be reasonable that Stephen does not invite friends to visit if he is living in his son's home or that Stephen may feel inclined to ask for permission to use the phone. However, it is less reasonable if Stephen owns the home and has assumed this kind of isolating behavior after his son has moved in with him. Home ownership is particularly important to evaluate in cases where an elderly person has remarried and now feels that he or she must seek permission to have reasonable use of the home and its amenities. Therefore, if the relative is a spouse, it is important to ascertain whether this is a second marriage, the length of marriage, and in whose home the individuals are residing.

Some useful questions to assist older victims in telling their story include the following:

- Does Al live with you in your home, or do you live in Al's home?
- I've seen other people with injuries like yours. How did this happen to you?
- When your son gets angry, how does he behave toward you?
- If you needed help because someone was violent in your home toward you, what would you do?
- Does someone in your family have power of attorney (or representative payee of Social Security)? What made you decide to give him or her that? Did you have your own attorney? Are you comfortable with your choice?
- Do you know how much money you have? Do you have access to your money whenever you want it?
- Are you ever afraid not to give your son money when he asks you for it? What would he do if you didn't give him the money he asked for?
- I see a lot of depressed people. Some of them are depressed because of their home situations, and how family members treat them. Tell me about your home and your family.
- Can you tell me how you are feeling right now?

Frank and Maria

Frank, 45 years old, lives with his 71 year-old mother, Maria. This admission to the county detoxification center was Frank's third. Maria was listed next of kin but never visited, because she did not drive. Therefore, she never attended any of the suggested family therapy sessions. At the end of each stay, the discharge planner made sure to inform Maria of her son's targeted discharge date, always asking if she had any questions. Maria's standard question was always the same: "Do you think he is ready to come home? Will he stop drinking now? Will he be able to hold a job now?" Frank was discharged to his mother's home as always.

In this case, examining the living situation may also give insights into the quality of the relationship between the elderly individual and relative. As indicated in Figure 7.2, Frank's mother Maria is a possible victim because of Frank's dependency for housing and his substance abuse history. Many relatives who move in with an older person have the best intentions, but others may do so because they have limited choices in their lives. When a relative moves in because of limited choices available (e.g., because of unemployment or eviction), the living situation becomes "forced" for both parties. Frank may not want to live with his mother, but because of his alcoholism and its effect on his ability to earn a living he has no other option. Maria may not want Frank living with her, particularly when he is actively drinking but feels that the situation is out of her control because

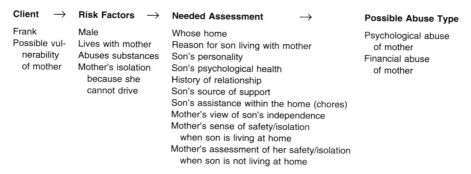

Client	→	Risk Factors	→	Needed Assessment	→	Possible Abuse Type
Frank		Male		Whose home		Psychological abuse
Possible vul-		Lives with mother		Reason for son living with mother		of mother
nerability		Abuses substances		Son's personality		Financial abuse
of mother		Mother's isolation		Son's psychological health		of mother
		because she		History of relationship		
		cannot drive		Son's source of support		
				Son's assistance within the home (chores)		
				Mother's view of son's independence		
				Mother's sense of safety/isolation		
				when son is living at home		
				Mother's assessment of her safety/isolation		
				when son is not living at home		

Figure 7.2. A case of possible financial abuse.

he does not move out when she asks him to leave. Frank may become extremely controlling of Maria to retain this living arrangement as an option. One means of control is isolating her from important social connections. Isolation of a victim is one of the primary risk factors in all forms of abuse. It is done so others will not notice the changes in the elderly person's lifestyle, and it gives the perpetrator more opportunity to control the elderly person's life. Engaging Maria in a telephone dialogue and asking her if she requested that Frank move in with her, and for what reason, may give some insight into this factor.

When the elderly person is not the client being serviced, as in the case of Frank and Maria, health care professionals may not aggressively pursue evaluating the in-home situation. The focus of treatment is on Frank, and because he is alert and competent, health care professionals may rely on him for validation of all discharge information. This can be further complicated by repeat admissions when the discharge plan has always been a return to the same living environment. In cases where clients may be difficult to place for discharge, whoever assumes responsibility for developing and executing the discharge plan may unwittingly support an inappropriate discharge to an older person's home. In Frank's case, if his need for housing and previous discharges to his mother's home; his history of chronic alcoholism, lack of income, and financial assets; Maria's lack of rapport with the treatment staff; and the community's lack of housing are all considered, then concern for Maria may indicate that she be actively engaged in a conversation to ascertain her concern for her safety. Therefore, in cases where it is impossible to interview the older person within the health facility environment, a person trained in telephone interviewing should evaluate any concerns the older person has in the continued provision of housing. Evaluating whether substance abuse or violence has ever been an issue in the relationship—and, if so, how it might have changed throughout the years—is helpful. Practitioners who assume that adult children—or hospitalized spouses, for that matter—are the providers of care within the home to older people, instead of assessing the actual provision of care, dependency issues, and quality of the relationship, may not recognize potential abusive situations. In this case, Frank also needed to be asked about how he helps around the house, how his mother's living space has changed since sharing occupancy, and if his mother tends to provide him with financial support. Some useful questions in this case scenario, which could be phrased for either Frank or Maria, would include the following:

- What sort of chores does Frank help you with around the house? What sort of chores do you wish he would do that he's not currently doing? Are you comfortable asking him for help?
- How have you changed your lifestyle since Frank has moved into your home? For example, have you stopped inviting friends over?
- You seem very worried about your son. Tell me about this worry.
- Are you sometimes frightened you will make Frank mad?
- How does he act when he doesn't drink? How about when he's had four drinks; how does he act?

Dorothy and Ed

Dorothy, 69 years of age, had a history of being seen at the local mental health clinic for depression. After being widowed for 5 years, she had recently remarried. The agency staff had not seen her for 4 years, but she was now seeking help because she was feeling depressed again. In the course of her treatment, she made passing remarks about not being sure she liked having sex with her new husband, Ed. She stated she had sex only so that he would stop "bothering her" but that it made her uncomfortable and that sometimes it hurt. She was verbally given some information about ways of making sexual contact more comfortable as well as a handout on sexual activity and the aged body. Her comments invoked little else in follow-up or concern, and she did not mention it again.

As illustrated in Figure 7.3, Dorothy represents a case of possible sexual abuse by her husband, who may feel that sexual intercourse is his prerogative because she is his wife. Or, her case may indicate a history of an abusive marital relationship. The first interesting feature of the case is the lack of concern of the therapist regarding the possible forced sexual advances of Dorothy's husband. Loue (2001) cited several reasons this omission may occur and stated that sexual abuse of elderly people is one of the more difficult forms to detect. Little is known about this phenomenon, because it has largely been ignored by the health and research communities; older people are "portrayed as having no interest in sex" (Loue, 2001, p. 164).

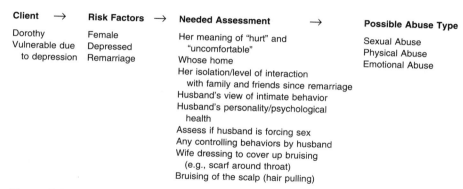

Client	→	Risk Factors	→	Needed Assessment	→	Possible Abuse Type
Dorothy Vulnerable due to depression		Female Depressed Remarriage		Her meaning of "hurt" and "uncomfortable" Whose home Her isolation/level of interaction with family and friends since remarriage Husband's view of intimate behavior Husband's personality/psychological health Assess if husband is forcing sex Any controlling behaviors by husband Wife dressing to cover up bruising (e.g., scarf around throat) Bruising of the scalp (hair pulling)		Sexual Abuse Physical Abuse Emotional Abuse

Figure 7.3. A case of possible sexual abuse.

Discussions of "sexuality in later life are often taboo" (Loue, 2001, p. 165). Feelings of shame or embarrassment may inhibit both perpetrator and victim and encourage them to deny it. Also, members of today's older generation have the social mores that sexual involvement outside of marriage was inappropriate (Loue, 2001). This case is further complicated by the fact that Dorothy was previously treated for depression. The clinician may be too dependent on past records to ascertain the current reasons for her depression, thereby not asking probing questions that would explore new triggers to her depressive episode. Issues of professional ageism may also be a factor in that older people are often seen as asexual, leading the clinician to assume that Dorothy's reluctance to have sexual relations is embedded in her lack of desire versus inappropriate behaviors of her new spouse. The following questions might be useful in helping the therapist examine if this is a case of suspected sexual abuse:

- You seem concerned about pleasing your husband. Do you sometimes find you do things you would rather not do to try to please him? What bothers you about doing that?
- Do you think it is the wife's duty to have sex with her husband when she doesn't want to have sex?
- When you say "It hurts me to have sex," what do you mean?
- Does your husband (partner) stop having sex with you when you tell him you're uncomfortable?
- Do you wish your husband would not have sex with you? How come?
- What is the best thing about your marriage, and what is the worst thing?
- Can you disagree with your husband? What happens when you do?

INTERVIEWING TO CONFIRM SUSPICION OF ABUSE

The phrasing of questions in the assessment process to confirm suspicion of abuse is important. Mental health counselors must be able to convey concern for the victim and, depending on the abuse category suspected, also for the relative thought to be the perpetrator of the suspected abuse. Because of the complexities of spousal and parent–adult child relationships, elderly people's suspicion of the mental health system, their concerns for losing control of decision making, and their fear that resolution of their abusive situation may be nursing home placement, the assessment process must be thorough, supportive, and reassuring (Schiamberg & Gans, 2000). It is important to inform elderly clients of the elder abuse reporting law; educate them about the protective system they may confront once a report is filed; and offer to assist them through the investigative process, if appropriate.

When interviewing suspected perpetrators it may also be important to express concern for their well-being, while being clear about the obligations of the elder abuse reporting law and communicating that any form of abuse is unacceptable. Suggesting to alleged perpetrators how to make their needs known through the investigative process for possible assistance is advisable.

Phrasing questions several different ways, asking same-theme questions several times, and using nonconfrontational questions mixed with indirect questions are all useful interview techniques (Welfel et al., 2000). Fearful elderly people will not admit to any form of abuse or neglect in front of the perpetrator; separate interviews allow each to tell his or her own story. Separate interviews may not be possible because of problems experienced by the older person (e.g., dementia, aphasia, hearing loss, or withdrawn personality) but should always be considered.

Caregivers may make very reasonable requests to be present with the older person to ensure that he or she fully expresses his or her concerns and that the professional fully understands what is troubling the older person and the scope of caregiving that the relative is attempting to provide. These caregivers should not be denied this opportunity; hence, conducting a joint interview, which also allows the professional to observe how caregiver and older person interact with each other, is useful. However, if possible, a separate interview should always follow this process.

CONCLUSION

Elder abuse is a form of family violence that can lead to illness, premature death, and dramatically decreased quality of life for older adults. Therefore, mental health practitioners must be prepared to know the various forms of abuse, assess all older people for abusive situations, understand the reporting laws in their states, acknowledge their obligation to report, and know how and where to make reports of suspected elder abuse (Bergeron & Gray, 2003; Freed & Drake, 1999). Mental health professionals should also learn about resources that are useful in understanding elder abuse, and ensure that professional training in all aspects of elder domestic violence becomes part of their continuing education.

Finally, mental health professionals need to communicate and form alliances with elderly and adult protective services practitioners. These practitioners have much to share with the mental health community about understanding elder abuse, interviewing suspected victims and perpetrators of elder abuse, and intervening in these situations. Conversely, the mental health community is a valuable resource to the elder abuse practitioners, because mental health practitioners often see older people at risk and have therapeutic strategies for intervening in situations involving substance and drug abuse, dysfunctional family relationships, personality disorders, and mental competency and mental health issues. Joining local multidisciplinary coalitions is a useful, efficient, and effective means by which to share expertise, develop respect for each other's professional talents, acquire educational forums, and present ethical and practice concerns. Elder abuse resources for mental health professionals to help accomplish these steps are listed at the end of this chapter.

The elder abuse literature contains little about effective therapeutic interventions for elderly victims. Interventions are needed that promote older people's acceptance of help, changing their enabling behaviors that may promote abuse, and helping them recognize their own self-worth so that they can let go of unhealthy relationships. Equally important are interventions for perpetrators of abuse. Researchers and practitioners need to develop case studies, assessment tools, treatment protocols, and outcome measures for elder abuse intervention that may be used across and within various disciplines.

Elder abuse is a growing problem in need of the same concern afforded to other forms of family violence. Mental health professionals can contribute to furthering the development of assessment, diagnostic, and intervention techniques for elderly victims, perpetrators of abusive action, and other family members who are involved with both victim and perpetrator.

ADDITIONAL RESOURCES

Clearinghouse on Abuse and Neglect of the Elderly (CANE), University of Delaware, Department of Consumer Studies, Alison Hall West, Room 211, Newark, DE 19716, 303-831-3525, CANE-UD@udel.edu

Goldman Institute on Aging's San Francisco, Consortium for Elder Abuse Prevention, 3330 Geary Boulevard, San Francisco, CA 94118, 415-750-4180

National Center on Elder Abuse (NCEA), 1225 I Street, NW, Suite 725, Washington, DC, 20005, 202-898-2586, http://www.elderabusecenter.org

National Committee for the Prevention of Elder Abuse, 1101 Vermont Avenue, NW, Suite 1001, Washington, DC, 20005, 202-682-4140, ncpea@erols.com, http://www.preventelderabuse.org

REFERENCES

Anetzberger, G. J. (2000). Caregiving: Primary cause of elder abuse? *Generations, 24*(2), 46–52.

Anetzberger, G. J. (2001). Elder abuse identification and referral: The importance of screening tools and referral protocols. *Journal of Elder Abuse & Neglect, 13*(2), 3–21.

Baron, S., & Welty, A. (1996). Elder abuse. *Journal of Gerontological Social Work, 25*(1/2), 33–57.

Bergeron, L. R. (2000). Servicing the needs of elder abuse victims. *Policy and Practice, 58*(3), 40–45.

Bergeron, L. R. (2001). An elder abuse case study: Caregiver stress or domestic violence? You decide. *Journal of Gerontological Social Work, 34*(4), 47–63.

Bergeron, L. R., & Gray, B. (2003). Ethical dilemmas of reporting suspected elder abuse. *Social Work, 48*, 96–105.

Brandl, B., & Raymond, J. (1997). Unrecognized elder abuse victims. *Journal of Case Management, 6*(2), 62–68.

Cyphers, G. C. (1999). Elder abuse and neglect. *Policy and Practice, 57*(3), 25–30.

Dunlop, B., Rothman, M., Condon, K., Hebert, K., & Martinez, I. (2000). Elder abuse: Risk factors and use of case data to improve policy and practice. *Journal of Elder Abuse and Neglect, 12*, 95–122.

Dyer, C. B., Pavlik, V. N., Murphy, K. P., & Hyman, D. J. (2000). The high prevalence of depression and dementia in elder abuse or neglect. *Journal of the American Geriatric Society, 48*, 205–208.

Ehrlich, R., & Anetzberger, G. (1991). Survey of state public health departments on procedures for reporting elder abuse. *Public Health Reports, 106*, 151–154.

Freed, P., & Drake, V. K. (1999). Mandatory reporting of abuse: Practical, moral, and legal issues for psychiatric home healthcare nurses. *Issues in Mental Health Nursing, 20*, 423–436.

Fulmer, T. (1991). Elder mistreatment: Progress in community detection and intervention. *Family and Community Health, 14*(2), 26–34.

Gerlock, A. (1999). Health impact of domestic violence. *Issues in Mental Health Nursing, 20*, 373–385.

Harris, S. (1996). For better or worse: Spouse abuse grown old. *Journal of Elder Abuse and Neglect, 8,* 1–33.

Jordan, L. C. (2001). Elder and domestic violence: Overlapping issues and legal remedies. *American Journal of Family Law, 15,* 147–156.

Kallman, H. (1987). Detecting abuse in the elderly. *Medical Aspects of Human Sexuality, 21*(3), 89–99.

Kosberg, J. I., & Garcia, J. L. (1995a). Common and unique themes on elder abuse from a world-wide perspective. *Journal of Elder Abuse and Neglect, 6*(3/4), 183–197.

Kosberg, J. I., & Garcia, J. L. (1995b). Introduction to the book. *Journal of Elder Abuse and Neglect, 6*(3/4), 1–12.

Krug, E., Mercy, J., Dahlberg, L., & Zwl, A. (2002). The world report on violence and health. *The Lancet, 360,* 1083–1088.

Lechner, V. M. (1993). Support systems and stress reduction among workers caring for dependent parents. *Social Work, 38,* 461–469.

Loue, S. (2001). Elder abuse and neglect in medicine and law. *Journal of Legal Medicine, 22,* 159–209.

National Elder Abuse Incidence Study. (1998). *Final report* (prepared for the Administration for Children and Families, and the Administration on Aging in the U.S., Department of Health and Human Services). Washington, DC: National Center on Elder Abuse.

Penhale, B. (1999). Bruises on the soul: Older women, domestic violence, and elder abuse. *Journal of Elder Abuse and Neglect, 11*(1), 1–22.

Peterson, M., & Paris, B. E. C. (1995). Elder abuse and neglect: How to recognize warning signs and intervene. *Geriatrics, 50*(4), 47–52.

Ramsey-Klawsnik, H. (2000). Elder abuse offenders: Types of offenders. Comparison of offenders. *Generations, 24*(2), 17–23.

Reis, M., & Nahmiash, D. (1997). Abuse of seniors: Personality, stress, and other indicators. *Journal of Mental Health and Aging, 3,* 337–356.

Schiamberg, L. B., & Gans, D. (2000). Elder abuse by adult children: An applied ecological framework for understanding contextual risk factors and the intergenerational character of quality of life. *International Journal of Aging and Human Development, 50,* 329–359.

Schneewind, E. (1994). Of ageism, suicide, and limiting life. *Journal of Gerontological Social Work, 23,* 135–150.

Seaver, C. (1996). Muted lives: Older battered women. *Journal of Elder Abuse and Neglect, 8*(2), 3–21.

Shock, L. P. (2000). Responding to evidence of abuse in the elderly. *Journal of the American Academy of Physician Assistants, 13*(6), 73–79.

Sijuwade, P. O. (1995). Cross-cultural perspectives on elder abuse as a family dilemma. *Social Behavior and Personality, 23,* 247–252.

Vinton, L. (1992). Battered women's shelters and older women: The Florida experience. *Journal of Family Violence, 7,* 63–72.

Welfel, E. R., Danzinger, P. R., & Santoro, S. (2000). Mandated reporting of abuse/maltreatment of older adults: A primer for counselors. *Journal of Counseling and Development, 78,* 284–293.

Wolf, R. S. (1996). Elder abuse and family violence: Testimony presented before the U.S. Senate special committee on aging. *Journal of Elder Abuse and Neglect, 8*(1), 81–96.

8

HEALTH CARE NEEDS OF ABUSE SURVIVORS AT MIDLIFE AND BEYOND

JANE RYSBERG

Recent research on aging Holocaust survivors indicates that those who experienced trauma in childhood or adolescence often have difficulties as they age. Yet less is known about elderly survivors of childhood abuse than almost any other victimized group. As the U.S. population ages, the needs of older abuse survivors will become more and more important. This chapter offers an exploratory look at the potential difficulties abuse survivors may face in midlife and old age. It describes normal developmental milestones and highlights how these events might be more difficult for people who have been abused earlier in their lives.

> Grow old along with me!
> The best is yet to be.
> —Robert Browning

Anyone who has read gerontology literature has encountered this phrase. Is it a promise? Can one outlive the effects of abuse? Is there a point in time when the existence of a childhood trauma can be ignored?

The scientific study of aging did not begin until the 1920s (Charles, 1970). Therefore, Robert Browning was speaking as a self-taught gerontologist with limited experience; he died at 68, and his wife, Elizabeth Barrett Browning, was only 51 when she died. The Brownings were, for their time, well read and well-known. They had access to adequate shelter, food, and health care. They spent much of their adult lives in temperate Italy, and they lived during a historical period when respect for older people was at least verbalized. These factors conform to some of those theorized to underlie optimal aging (e.g., Baltes & Reichert, 1992). If one defines the "best" as a point in an individual's life when psychological maturity and possibly happiness are present, then the later years might be golden (Sheldon & Kasser, 2001).

If one asked an elderly individual today if she were experiencing her later years as the best part of her life, how would she respond? The specific answer is impossible to predict. However, one can identify older people who would be more likely to respond with "no". An elderly woman who is impoverished and has few educational, economic, and social resources is likely to rate her health as poor. She is also likely to have low life satisfaction and poor self-efficacy. If she acknowledged, or one suspected, a history of abuse, her health and other age-related problems would be likely to be exaggerated. For example, a sequela of abuse is often depression. Depression in an older person often mimics certain aspects of dementia. A history of depression may have shaped her lifestyle choices, so that she may have abused drugs, eaten poorly, and lived in isolation for significant periods in her young and middle adulthood. She now displays hypertension and sleep disorders; is underweight; and suffers from arthritis, which she describes as causing excruciating pain. She forgets to take prescribed medications, and she misses appointments.

What would be an acceptable and realistic recovery goal for this client? Treatment for depression could modify the apparent cognitive decline and improve the client's participation in treatment and self-care. It is possible that some physical symptoms were related to the depression; an elderly client may find it more acceptable to talk about physical health than mental health. Improvements in mobility, mood tone, appetite, and sleep patterns could follow from a multifaceted approach to the client's symptoms. Improvement in a client's rating of his or her own physical health is often associated with an increase in life satisfaction in the elderly adult. To understand and anticipate the treatment needs of elderly abuse survivors, medical and mental health professionals need a grasp on the normative experience of aging. This is described in the next section.

THE EXPERIENCE OF AGING

When one looks at the aging process in a given elderly person, there are three major categories of influences that must be examined. The first are called *normative age-graded influences*. Developmental psychologists have studied this category intensively because of its universal nature. Normative age-graded influences are biological and social and are highly correlated with chronological age. Examples are timing of first marriage, entrance into the workforce, menopause, graying of hair, and the acquisition of bifocals. The second category, *normative history-graded influences*, happen to a population of people at a given point in time. They are events such as plague, war, or recession. The third category of influences is called *non-normative*. They are not experienced by everyone but can be very significant. A person may be elected president, lose a limb in a car accident, or be abused as a child or adult.

Manifestations of normative age-graded influences are eagerly awaited during the early developmental periods. Children are thrilled with a new tooth, and their parents are impressed with the advance represented by the acquisition of the pincer grasp. These biological events are called *developmental milestones*. Adults of middle age and beyond may experience normative age-graded events as "milestones," "transitions," or "crises," depending on the individual. Gerontologists prefer to call them *influences*. These influences are typically anticipated and are often objects of preparation. The manifestations may be met with a range of emotions and may occur over a prolonged period. They occur within the family, in the workplace, and within the adult.

Family Events

The family milestones of middle and late adulthood are as follows.

- *Launching of children.* This commences with children's movement out of the home and includes events such as mate selection and the birth of grandchildren.
- *Changing relationship with family members of the preceding generation.* How do your in-laws intend to handle their retirement, socially and economically? Are your parents becoming more frail?
- *Possible changes in the marital union.* Changes in the marital union include dissolution, remarriage, or loss of companionship due to the onset of Alzheimer's disease in the spouse.

Unlike the acquisitions of developmental milestones in early childhood, the specific context of these changes can be very important. The middle-class parents who are helping their college-graduate son move from home to a lovely new apartment near his first job are having very different feelings from the parents whose 17-year-old son abandoned the family home after a series of fights with Dad. Yet both sets of parents would be described as being engaged in "launching" activities.

Milestones in the Workforce

Most people residing in America today have an expectation that they will work outside of the home for at least some portion of their lives. The ideal work life envisioned by Americans is a long, stable one, crowned with retirement (Hayward, Friedman, & Chen, 1998). In certain sectors of the economy, older workers may be selectively more likely to be in older businesses. Therefore they experience a disproportionate share of job changes. There appears to be little age-related decline in many job categories, and the productivity of older workers is on a par with that of younger workers (Warr, 1998). However, an elderly person who loses a job will be unlikely to find a new job commensurate with the old one (Gardner, 1995).

Retirement may mean a long-anticipated and voluntary movement out of the workforce, or it may be the result of an inability to find a job after a lengthy search. It can mean an opportunity to try new activities at a leisurely pace, or it can mean a descent into poverty. Even if retirement was planned, one can debate the meaning of this event in a nation such as the United States, where we introduce ourselves as "Bob Smith, Banker."

Intra-Individual Milestones

People attend all of the important events in the workplace, and with their families, wearing their bodies. Most people act as if the most salient hallmark of increasing years on the planet is a changing body. In addition, many of these people would indicate that these changes in the body represent declines. If one asked a random selection of Americans to pick out the older people in a group, they would probably search for gray hairs and wrinkles rather than a right arm made strong by 50 years of work, fly fishing, and picking up babies.

The longest known life span is that of Jeanne Calmet, who died in 1997 at the age of 122. That is an admirable life span; however, many people are aware of the maxim that it is not the "years in our life, but the life in our years." According to the National Center for Health Statistics (1998), the life expectancy of a child born today (i.e., as this chapter is being written) is approximately 76 years. Starting at about age 40, this person will become aware of impactful changes in the body. These changes may be age related.

There are three types of age-related changes, called *primary, secondary,* and *tertiary* aging. Primary aging is the result of normal changes that occur during adulthood. Menopause and changes in the eye that result in increasing far-sightedness are examples. Primary aging is universal. Secondary aging occurs with increasing time on the earth and is displayed in huge numbers of adults, yet these changes are not inevitable. Secondary aging is the result of disease, disuse, or abuse. Loss of cognitive abilities is not "natural" or universal, so dementia is a result of secondary aging. Decline in auditory acuity after several decades in an environment with heavy noise pollution is another example. The rapid losses that occur right before death are called tertiary aging.

Neurological Changes

If one starts at the top of the head of a potential elderly client, one can observe typical bodily changes. It appears that the loss of some neurons and neuronal structures is found over time even in healthy people, with the appearance of significant numbers of new dendrites and synapses also possible (Scheibel, 1996). Changes in the brain's structure and functioning might be expected to correlate with changes in behavior. Older people are more likely to indicate that they have difficulty falling asleep and staying asleep, and that they have poor-quality sleep, than are younger adults (Whitbourne, 1999). They also have difficulty telling when their core body temperature is low, or responding, behaviorally or physiologically, when the temperature is very high (Besdine, 1995).

Visual Changes

Normal changes in the lens, the retina, and the eye muscles, combined with conditions such as cataracts and glaucoma, mean that most older people experience some degree of visual impairment. Eyeglasses might be considered part of the "uniform" of the elderly population. The degree of impairment and an individual's ability to obtain treatment means the difference between telling jokes about one's ever-shortening arms and experiencing social isolation because one has been forced to give up driving.

Auditory Changes

Auditory impairments follow a developmental path similar to that of visual impairment, with persons between age 40 and 70 being increasingly likely to complain of problems. The use of language is an important part of one's daily life; therefore, a decline in one's ability to hear speech clearly is a significant problem. As with vision, there are methods of remediation, the most common being the hearing aid. Many adults are willing to wear glasses, but far fewer are willing to use a hearing aid, possibly because the aid does not always improve the clarity and comprehension of speech sounds. Hearing aids can be dispensed by salespersons who are not qualified audiologists. Even a well-fitted hearing aid can have significant drawbacks, such as amplifying background noise just as much as conversation. The use of a hearing aid has not been found to necessarily increase social activities or satisfaction with social relations (Tesch-Romer, 1997).

Other Sensory Changes

Just as vision and audition have a downward progression with age, could one expect that all of the other senses would decline as well? One can imagine that declines in the sensitivity to odors and tastes would diminish life's pleasures. Taste and smell acuity appear to decline slightly, although older people may not be too aware of the loss (Nordine, Monsch, & Murphy, 1995). One might also expect that a decline in sensitivity to pain would be a boon. The outcome of research on the decline of pain thresholds is inconsistent: The outcomes are confounded with type of pain, location of pain, who is experiencing the pain, and the management of the pain (Wisocki & Powers, 1997).

Change in the sense of *kinesthesis*, or awareness of bodily positions, movements, and tensions, is associated with changes in other senses. Elderly people often have concerns about being unsteady on their feet and taking a tumble. This loss of balance can be tied to the decline in visual acuity, changes in the vestibular system, and a brain that integrates sensory information more slowly than in its younger days (Whitbourne, 1999). Older people's fear of falling is real, as one is more likely to experience a fall, and to be harmed in the fall, as one moves into the seventh decade (Whitbourne, 1999).

Declines in the senses occur very gradually, so most adults do not notice the losses until the late 40s. This slow decrement allows people to gradually adjust to some of the changes without much awareness. The typical older adult can still perform the basic activities of daily living with diminished hearing, vision, and postural control. Daily tasks become more difficult when the burden of chronic and acute diseases are added.

Changes in Health

The National Center for Health Statistics (1999) estimated that evidence of at least one form of arthritis can be found in every American over the age of 60, with the majority feeling some pain from the disease. Some older people regard the original aches and pains indicating arthritis as inevitable and so do not seek treatment. Even without treatment, however, people do not die of this disease. The number one cause of death for adults is heart disease. The most common reason for hospitalization for individuals over the age of 65 is congestive heart failure. A myocardial infarction is more likely to be lethal for an older adult than a younger one. Some of the pathways to heart disease involve factors under a person's control, whereas others involve genetic, gender, and age factors (American Heart Association, 1998). Over time, the walls of the arteries become calcified, meaning that they are less elastic. The heart muscle, including valves, also becomes stiffer, resulting in less blood being moved per minute. If fat deposits are added to the artery walls, and the blood supply to the brain is reduced, one has the introduction of another condition: cerebrovascular disease. Complete loss of the blood supply to a particular portion of the brain results in a *cerebrovascular accident*, commonly referred to as a *stroke*. The likelihood that one will recover from a stroke depends on the brain area affected, the extent and duration of the loss of the blood supply, and the age at the time of the stroke. The risk of stroke increases with age, so that stroke is a common cause of death for older people.

How do older adults feel about their aging bodies? When interviewed, older adults mention chronic health problems such as hypertension more frequently than do younger or middle-aged adults. This doubtless contributes to the existence of more significant health-related stress in older people (Wrosch, Heckhausen, & Lachman, 2000).

Acknowledging Variability Among Older People

One can look at "typical" aging. One cannot, however, find a "typical" adult, as variability is a key concept of the aging process. Individual genotypes are acted on by a wide array of physical, psychological, and social environments. Adults further increase the diversity of their experiences by interpreting them in a variety of ways. For example, one woman may believe that her single marital status at age 50 is an opportunity for personal growth, whereas another may perceive her failure to marry as a sentence to social isolation. Some theorists (e.g., Thomae, 1990, speaking specifically on personality development) have gone so far as to argue that individual differences in aging are so wide that there are no general rules. Some attempts to explain the experience of aging—for example, branching theory (Schroots, 1996)—predict quality of life, mortality, and morbidity as the result of choices of higher or lower levels of functioning in biological, social, and psychological realms. This type of theory has parallels in the contemporary study of physics, where it is called *chaos theory*. Both in physics and in psychology, these types of theories predict that systems will tend to disorganization prior to the demise of the system.

Mental health practitioners who take the opportunity to work with older people must acknowledge the great variation among this client population. They will observe that events of aging that leave physical traces provide clinicians with an entry point into a particular older adult's experiences. They may ask "How do you feel about your loss of mobility? How can we help you cope with this change?" Elderly people are generally good assessors of their own health status (Pinquart, 2001).

Is abuse a life experience that alters the body? How might trauma interact with the process of aging? Where should the practitioner look? Social scientists first search the literature. There are few studies of the long-term mental and physical health needs of older abuse survivors. One must look for hints.

THE INTERSECTION OF AGING AND CHILDHOOD TRAUMA

A recent *Harvard Heart Letter* (2001) asked a provocative question: Will there be an increase in deaths over the next few months of adults who lost loved ones in the September 11 attacks on the World Trade Center? The mechanism that could account for this increase in mortality would be a change in hormonal activities, triggering potentially harmful changes in blood pressure, immune cells, and heart rate.

It is known that long-term negative emotions are associated with negative health outcomes. During the 1960s, researchers began using the Minnesota Multiphasic Personality Inventory (Hathaway & McKinley, 1989) to group people according to their tendency to predict negative outcomes and to assume blame for these unhappy events. Followed for 30 years, people with a negative outlook were more likely to have made greater use of both mental and physical health services. Their death rate was higher than that of same-age participants who displayed more positive emotions (Maruta, Colligan, Malinchoc, & Offord, 2000). Are people with a negative outlook more likely to dismiss medical advice, or does a negative outlook stress the physical system? What if a person's life experiences led him or her to believe that the worst was likely to happen *and* significant stress had damaged aspects of the physiological system? What if these harmful physical and psychological changes acted on a body that was also compromised by age-related declines?

Findings From Aging Holocaust Survivors

A history of trauma is an example of a negative, non-normative life event. Do events of this type encompass changes to both the body and the mind? Solomon and Ginzburg (1998, 1999) have examined the literature and conducted research on the impact of previous trauma on the adjustment to aging. They concluded that there are clear differences between elderly individuals who experienced early trauma and those who did not. These differences appeared both in adjustment to aging and in reactions to subsequent stressors. Earlier in their lives, the Holocaust survivors did well. However, they started to experience difficulties as they became less "busy" and as they hit the milestones of middle and old age. Retirement was often difficult, as were times of illness and hospitalization and when children left home.

Solomon and Ginzburg (1998, 1999) also have studied these differences in samples of residents of Israel during the Gulf War. Although all of their participants were older, only a portion were survivors of the Holocaust. Significantly more Holocaust survivors reported experiencing psychological distress; anxiety; problems in cognitive activities, such as concentration and memory; and loss of interest in significant others and activities. Also more frequent were reports of physical changes, such as sleep disorders and irritability. Solomon and Ginzburg checked for possible confounding factors, such as gender, and found that the differences between Holocaust survivors and others remained robust.

Negative Life Events Among Elderly People

Both the Gulf War and the Holocaust are unique historical events. Israel is a unique environment. Do Solomon and Ginzburg's (1998, 1999) findings apply to other participants and other types of trauma? De Kraaij (2001) investigated the impact of negative life events in an elderly community sample. *Negative life events* were defined as experiences such as neglect, sexual or emotional abuse during childhood, problems in a significant relationship, poor socioeconomic conditions, or sexual or emotional abuse during adulthood. Depression in late adulthood was related to the experience of negative life events. Depression was deepened if multiple negative events were experienced and if more of the events occurred in childhood. Although they sampled different populations and used different examples of trauma, both Solomon and Ginzburg (1998, 1999) and de Kraaij (2001) concluded that clinicians must be vigilant. They encouraged clinicians to seek specific information from their elderly clients about their history with traumatic events. The information sought should include the client's response to the original event and to subsequent stressful events.

Harel (1995) also looked at the clinical needs of Holocaust survivors. While generally concurring with the suggestions of de Kraaij (2001) and Solomon and Ginzburg (1998, 1999), Harel provided additional components of appropriate clinical interventions for trauma survivors. While survivors were potentially accumulating experiences of extreme stress, they were also aging. Therefore, their adjustment to aging needed to be examined, with an emphasis on their practiced coping strategies and the availability of coping resources. Coping strategies that had been serviceable in middle age, but were dependent on a circle of age mate supporters, might not be effective in the later years, when one's ranks of supporters have been thinned by death, dementia, or distance.

These warnings are important for the creation of appropriate behavioral supports and interventions with elderly people. However, clinicians also need to know how the continuing effects of early trauma are being transmitted. In addition, are there other aspects of the aging experience that may have been influenced by early exposure to traumatic events such as abuse?

Trauma and Long-Term Mental Health Status

It has long been suspected that abuse significantly alters the long-term mental health status of victims. Banyard, Williams, and Siegel (2001) analyzed the data collected from adult women participating in a longitudinal investigation on the consequences of childhood sexual abuse. In this ongoing study, survivors typically reported multiple episodes of trauma and multiple mental health symptoms. Banyard et al. concluded that early trauma can have both direct and indirect effects on adult development. In addition, they surmised that exposures to trauma are interconnected. Thus, the reactions of a young victim of sexual abuse may influence his or her reactions as an older trauma survivor. Is the relation between earlier and later reactions a result of learning? It would not be surprising if a child learned to distrust powerful adults in her life if she had been sexually abused by a person who should have been a loving caretaker. A generalization of this distrust to workplace peers could make an adult survivor appear to be paranoid. This seeming paranoia might contribute to significant emotional displays in the face of moderate stressors in daily life. It is important to look at the behavior of adult survivors, but it is not enough.

When working with adult clients with a variety of psychiatric disorders, contemporary practitioners may look for mind–body interactions. But where should they look? People seldom speak of an anxious elbow but often seek remedies for a nervous stomach and tension headaches. Using data from the Epidemiologic Catchment Area Project, North, Alpers, Thompson, and Spitznagel (1996) demonstrated that members of the general community who reported two or more undiagnosed gastrointestinal symptoms, such as abdominal pain, were also likely to display psychiatric symptoms. The incidence of long-term gastrointestinal symptoms was also highly correlated with long-term psychiatric disorders. This was an important study in that it demonstrated that the high incidence of psychiatric disorders found in patients visiting doctors' offices for treatment of functional bowel disorders was observable in a community sample. It was unfortunately not possible to determine whether the gastrointestinal problem predated the psychiatric problem, or vice versa.

After reviewing the literature on traumatic brain injury (TBI), van Reekum, Cohen, and Wong (2000) concluded that there was an association between TBI and some categories of psychiatric disorders. They concluded that TBI was not significantly related to either schizophrenia or substance abuse but that mood and anxiety disorders did seem to be strongly associated with TBI.

Silver, Kramer, Greenwald, and Weissman (2001) also used data from the Epidemiologic Catchment Area Project; they examined information from participants who reported head injuries. In this community sample, a head injury that resulted in a loss of consciousness or confusion was much more likely to be reported by adults with a range of psychiatric difficulties. These psychiatric problems included depression, suicide attempts, drug and alcohol abuse, and panic and phobic disorders. The authors controlled for relevant sociodemographic factors, such as educational level, and found that a poorer quality of life was also a long-term experience of head trauma victims.

A study of 1,718 veterans of World War II confirmed the presence of depression in individuals who had suffered previous trauma to the head (Holsinger et al., 2002). The researchers were able to examine the impact of injury severity and the timing of injuries. They found that loss of consciousness for a day or longer was more associated with depression than was a loss of consciousness for 30 or fewer minutes. In addition, the risk for depression after head injury was still present after as much as 50 years. Holsinger et al. concluded that a psychiatric disorder, such as depression, would be a cause for a recruit to be rejected for military service. They therefore posited that the head injury was the source of the depression.

The article, published in the *Archives of General Psychiatry* (Holsinger et al., 2002), was accompanied by an editorial arguing that this information on the long-term significance of head injuries should promote better care for victims of concussions. What should be the focus of this improvement in care? Should there be greater attention to the possible damage to the brain? Should victims of head trauma be provided with tools to cope with possible future bouts of depression? Or must attention be paid both to possible present changes in physiology and to associated changes in behavior?

CONCLUSION

An examination of recent research shows that trauma is associated with both physiological and behavioral changes. The underlying physiological changes, particularly changes in the structure and functioning of the brain, ensure that the body carries the information about past trauma into future stressful situations. It also ensures that traumatic changes in physiology can be acted on by the forces of physical aging. Basic laws of biology suggest that damaged cells and organ systems can function in ways to damage other cells or systems. The damage can cause negative changes in behavior, which can exacerbate the physiological problems. While recognizing the long-term impact of trauma, a therapist must recognize that the client is also involved in the process of adjusting to aging. In the next section I offer some specific suggestions about what psychologists can do to help aging abuse survivors deal with both the effects of aging and the long-term effects of trauma. Additional resources are included at the end of the chapter.

Clinical Intervention

In attempting to determine what is associated with successful aging, psychologists often look at behaviors that are thought to be under a person's control, such as attitudes and environments: beliefs in one's ability to seize the day and the role of friends. It has repeatedly been observed that one should be optimistic, take control, and have social relationships.

In a study, elderly Australian men who had experienced economic losses, declines in health, a loss of work, or some combination of these, experienced a reduction in well-being. Men who were mentally involved with personally satisfying activities, such as hobbies or community affairs, were more likely to be able to accept the losses and maintain positive adjustment to aging. This meant that subjective labels for events in the world were more important than the objective factors (Bar-Tur, Levy-Shiff, & Burns, 1998). Does this finding represent events found in a single slice of life, or does it point to relationships that could occur over considerable amounts of time?

Predispositions to respond in particular ways can be very durable. The "expected unchangeability of life stress" (EU) was best predicted by an older person's level of life satisfaction rather than by the presence or absence of economic or health problems (Thomae, 1981). An elderly person who had a high EU score identified more problematic behaviors as responses to stress. This pattern of responding may ensure that life stresses will continue at a consistent level. Adjustment to stressful situations in aging was better predicted by use of cognitive reappraisals (Thomae, 1981). Stressed elderly people may benefit from the creation of psychoeducational events that can assist them in reframing some of life's events.

Taking Control

Prenda and Lachman (2001) studied the relation between life satisfaction and perceptions of control. Who plans, and how they plan, were central questions in their research. Although the youngest participants were found to be the most planful, the correlation between life satisfaction and strategizing about the future was found to be the strongest for the older adults. This led Prenda and Lachman to recommend that caregivers and therapists encourage older people to plan their futures, as a way to increase life satisfaction and feelings of being in control.

Elderly trauma survivors could not control the abuse that was inflicted on them. This created stress at the time of the negative life event. Growing old in an ageist society such as that of the United States may provide new and unavoidable stressors. Because they may be physiologically predisposed to overreact to stressors, elderly trauma survivors may benefit from specific education on the introduction of new coping strategies. Situational reappraisal may be particularly effective. Past research (e.g., Prenda & Lachman, 2001) suggests that people do not automatically develop successful coping strategies simply by remaining on the planet for a significant number of years but that they can learn if they are specifically taught.

Go Through Life in a Convoy

Women make up the majority of research participants when successful aging is examined among the old-old (i.e., those over 85 years of age). Laferriere and Hamel-Bissell (1994) used interviews and observations to investigate the histories and contemporary experiences of very elderly women in rural New England. They concluded that successful aging was possible, even in the presence of chronic health problems, if a strong social network was in place.

What defines a strong social support network? The psychological and physical well-being of aging mothers of retarded adult children was examined by Hong, Seltzer, and Krauss (2001). For mothers over the age of 65, well-being was associated with the level of emotional support, not the size of the social network. A few well-chosen supporters were more effective than a loose crowd of contacts. It also looks as if it is possible to purposely build emotional support. An important source of emotional support was a plan for the continued guardianship of the retarded adult.

Social networks can have a prolonged history. People in need often look to friends and family members who provided succor in the past. Bumagin (1982) noted that family support tends to persist even when the construction of the family changes; widows and divorcees can count on more family support than can never-married women. People who were previously successful in relationships obtain more support than those who were not. This support can arise from the ties that were formed in the past, but previously successful women also show an ability to adapt to changes.

Suitor and Pillemer (2000) found that social support need not be long term in nature to be effective. In their Peer Support Project, the key to effectiveness was availability and experience. Could a new acquaintance make regular visits, and did the peer have experiences that could be beneficial in this situation?

Social support is important to positive adjustment to aging. The social support networks of elderly trauma survivors should be examined. If no supportive network exists, or if the existing network provides inadequate emotional support, a therapist may want to consider whether one can be built. Previous research suggests that even formal ties can be effective. Teaching elderly people to reach out to potential supporters may also be useful.

Assessment

Practitioners must obtain information about the elderly person's past as well as the present. It would be desirable if all elderly clients came to therapy with detailed medical records. This is not always possible, as many older people have been peripatetic. Even if they were relatively stationary, they may not have had a durable relationship with a physician. The only method of obtaining a life history may be from the individual him- or herself. The veracity of the life history may be affected by the elderly person's ability or desire to remember.

Assessments of an elderly person's functioning should be gathered in at least three major areas: (a) the tasks of daily living, (b) cognition, and (c) mood. The forms of assessment can range from informal conversations with observations made of the personal appearance and interpersonal interactions of the elderly client to formal intelligence testing with, for example (Luszcz, Bryan, & Kent, 1997), the Wechsler Adult Intelligence Scale—Revised (Wechsler, 1975), the Mini-Mental State Examination (Folstein, Folstein, & McHugh, 1975), or the National Adult Reading Test (Nelson & Willison, 1991).

An important piece of information about the present is how the older person feels about the process of aging. Is he or she satisfied with this period in life or experiencing anger and hostility? Several formal assessment instruments are available. An example is the Philadelphia Geriatric Center Morale Scale (Lawton, 1975) and the Life Satisfaction Index (Wood, Wylie, & Sheafor, 1969). This instrument has the advantage of being unaffected by the elderly person's level of activity (Filsinger & Sauer, 1978).

Possible Problems in the Therapeutic Situations

Providers may be part of the problem rather than part of the solution. James and Haley (1995) surveyed psychologists trained at the doctoral level. When faced with older and younger clients with the same presenting symptoms, practitioners consistently rated the prognosis for the older people as poorer. In addition, clients who had health problems were rated as having more psychological problems than were healthy individuals.

Having, or being perceived as having, more difficulties, may cause older people to experience additional problems. Preville, Herbert, Boyer, and Bravo (2001) examined the data from the Quebec Health Survey (1992–1993) using a multivariate logistic regression analysis. Twenty-two percent of elderly respondents had used a psychotropic medication in the 48 hr preceding data collection, compared with 4.9% of adults under the age of 64. When physical status was controlled, healthy elderly people were 7.49 times more likely to have prescriptions for psychotropic drugs than were healthy young adults. It appears that prescriptions are determined not only by physical conditions but also by a patient's characteristics.

Because older abuse victims may be more likely to have more health problems, providers must continuously remind themselves that treatment is appropriate and that success is possible. Another characteristic worthy of consideration is the complexity of an elderly client. Gottesman (2001), although writing specifically about a life span approach to genetic disorders such as schizophrenia, urged psychologists to accept probabilism as a philosophy in the face of complex psychopathologies. He pointed out that this perspective has brought success to the examination of the complex systems that combine to produce coronary artery disease. Therefore, practitioners must avoid assuming that an elderly abuse victim represents a specific constellation of problems and practitioners should be willing to work with possibilities.

There are no specific studies on abuse victims' adjustment to aging. It could be logical to assume that adjustment issues are present. Abuse victims who are elderly today may have experienced feelings of isolation, humiliation, and poor social relations arising from U.S. society's unwillingness to acknowledge and deal with the problem. This lack of social awareness and support was also experienced by both deaf and gay people who are elderly today. In spite of these historical difficulties, some elderly deaf people (Tidball, 1990), and some elderly gay men and lesbians (Adelman, 1990), have been found to have appropriate coping strategies and adjustment to aging. This type of variability might be present in elderly trauma survivors.

Selection of a Therapeutic Philosophy

When faced with an older client who has experienced abuse, a practitioner should acknowledge that the past trauma may underlie chronic health difficulties, social problems, and apparent difficulty adjusting to the aging process. This could lead to interventions focused on the past as well as on the present. In her model for assisting trauma survivors, Hanscom (2001) pointed out that the therapist needs to hear the history of the survivor, focusing on the emotions and reactions. It is also critical to ask about and explain the reasons for the physical and psychological symptoms. Teaching relaxation and coping strategies, and other forms of self-change, might seem like the outcome of the hearing and explaining; however, these components of treatment can occur in any order. Control and a future orientation are correlated with positive outcomes for older people; thus, it may be very important that elderly trauma victims guide the process of the therapy to help them gain a feeling of power over the past and the present.

How Can Services to Elderly Trauma Survivors Be Improved?

No longitudinal studies have examined how survivors of trauma age. Studies of tiny slices of the posttrauma lives of survivors are beginning to emerge. What are some of the pressing questions that, if answered, could improve clinical practices?

Information on diversity is needed. There is a growing body of literature on the experience of aging as a member of a minority group in America. The first observation is that members of minority groups have a shorter life expectancy than do White Americans. America is "graying," but the average life expectancy for an African American male is only 67.2 years, compared with the Caucasian male's 73.6 years (Hoyert, Kochaneck, & Murphy, 1999). Clark, Anderson, Clark, and Williams (1999) argued that stress is created by the experience, or the perception of the experience, of racism. Their biopsychosocial model delineates how this stress can affect health outcomes. Medical and mental health practitioners need to know how elderly Black trauma survivors are affected by the combination of racism and ageism. Were they less likely to receive services at the time of abuse? Were they less likely to be aware of support services to deal with the aftermath of abuse? If they received services at any point, were these services appropriate to their worldview?

Information also is needed on the interaction of the kinds of physiological changes that have been found in trauma survivors and secondary aging. What is the consequence of several decades of chronic hyperarousal? What kinds of changes will appear in an elderly brain that has been repeatedly bathed in stress hormones? In what kinds of self-medication might an older person have engaged to deal with chronic hyperarousal? How did these lifestyle decisions affect his or her secondary aging? Do the effects continue to accrue as the elderly person moves from the status of the young-old (i.e., persons from 65 on) to the status of old-old? Are there differences in dealing with end-of-life issues with elderly individuals whose health has been altered by the experience of abuse?

It has been assumed that clients who experienced abuse during childhood or adolescence were aware of their victimization. What if this is not true, or at least not completely true? Delayed-discovery statutes of limitations allow the legal clock to begin ticking when a person becomes aware of the injuries. What could be the progress of an elderly client who becomes aware of abuse during therapy for problems in adjustment to aging?

Finally, will the most appropriate forms of therapeutic intervention for aging survivors of abuse emphasize recovery from trauma or emphasize adjustment to aging? Is it possible that a hybrid of the two therapeutic forms will emerge?

In 1982, 26.2% of Americans over the age of 65 had a chronic disability. In 1999, this figure had shrunk to 19.7%. This suggests that recent advances in health care may be bringing closer to reality Browning's notion that the best period of life is its penultimate one. A review of the literature suggests that there are many more advances to be made, particularly in the area of care for traumatized elderly people.

An end to abuse does not mean an end to trauma. There are many ways in which negative effects can be perpetuated. Psychologists need to become more aware of the possible interactions between the consequences of abuse and the processes of primary and secondary aging.

Practitioners must also abandon the belief that an old dog cannot be taught any new tricks. Advances in assessment techniques and therapeutic interventions that address physical, cognitive, behavioral, and social aspects of the lives of elderly survivors of abuse are possible and necessary.

ADDITIONAL RESOURCES

Brown University Geriatric Psychopharmacology Update. Contains updates on the use of psychotropic medications in geriatrics and pertinent regulatory issues. http://www.medscape.com/psychiatry

Rowe, J. W., & Kahn, R. L. (1998). *Successful aging*. New York: Pantheon Books.

Zarit, S. H., & Knight, B. G. (Eds.). (1996). *A guide to psychotherapy and aging: Effective clinical interventions in a life-stage context*. Washington, DC: American Psychological Association.

REFERENCES

Adelman, M. (1990). Stigma, gay lifestyles and the adjustment to aging: A study of later-life gay men and lesbians. *Journal of Homosexuality, 20*, 7–32.

American Heart Association. (1998). *1999 heart and stroke statistical update*. Dallas, TX: Author.

Baltes, M. M., & Reichert, M. (1992). Successful aging: The product of biological factors, environmental quality and behavioral competence. In J. George & S. Ebrahim (Eds.), *Healthcare for older women* (pp. 236–256). Oxford, England: Oxford University Press.

Banyard, V. L., Williams, L. M., & Siegel, J. A. (2001). The long-term mental health consequences of child sexual abuse: An exploratory study of the impact of multiple traumas in a sample of women. *Journal of Traumatic Stress, 14,* 697–715.

Bar-Tur, L., Levy-Shiff, R., & Burns, A. (1998). Well-being in aging: Mental engagements in elderly men as a moderator of losses. *Journal of Aging Studies, 12,* 1–20.

Besdine, R. W. (1995). Hyperthermia and accidental hypothermia. In W. B. Abrams, M. H. Beers, & R. Berkow (Eds.), *The Merck manual of geriatrics* (2nd ed., pp. 47–57). Whitehouse Station, NJ: Merck Research Laboratories.

Bumagin, V. E. (1982). Growing old female. *Journal of Psychiatric Treatment and Evaluation, 4,* 155–159.

Charles, D. C. (1970). Historical antecedents of life-span developmental psychology. In L. R. Goulet & P. B. Baltes (Eds.), *Life-span developmental psychology: Research and theory* (pp. 24–53). New York: Academic Press.

Clark, R., Anderson, N. B., Clark, V. R., & Williams, D. R. (1999). Racism as a stressor for African Americans: A biopsychosocial model. *American Psychologist, 54,* 805–816.

Filsinger, E., & Sauer, W. J. (1978). An empirical typology of adjustment to aging. *Journal of Gerontology, 33,* 437–445.

Folstein, M. F., Folstein, S. E., & McHugh, P. R. (1975). Mini-mental state: A practical method for grading the cognitive state of patients for the clinician. *Journal of Psychiatric Research, 12,* 189–198.

Gardner, J. (1995, April). Worker displacement: A decade of change. *Monthly Labor Review,* 45–57.

Gottesman, I. I. (2001). Psychopathology through a life span–genetic prism. *American Psychologist, 56,* 867–878.

Hanscom, K. L. (2001). Treating survivors of war trauma and torture. *American Psychologist, 56,* 1032–1039.

Harel, Z. (1995). Serving Holocaust survivors and survivor families. *Marriage and Family Review, 21,* 29–49.

Harvard Heart Letter. (December 31, 2001). Can you die of a broken heart? Retrieved June 26, 2003, from http://www.hmiworld.org/past_issues/March_April_2002/broken_heart.html

Hathaway, S. R., & McKinley, J. C. (1989). *The Minnesota Multiphasic Personality Inventory-2.* Minneapolis: University of Minnesota Press.

Hayward, M. D., Friedman, S., & Chen, H. (1998). Career trajectories and older men's retirement. *Journal of Gerontology: Social Sciences, 53,* 91–103.

Holsinger, T., Steffens, D. C., Phillips, C., Helms, M. J., Havlik, R. J., Breitner, J. C. S., et al. (2002). Head injury in early adulthood and the lifetime risk of depression. *Archives of General Psychiatry, 59,*(1,) 17–22.

Hong, J., Seltzer, M. M., & Krauss, M. W. (2001). Change in social support and psychological well being: A longitudinal study of aging mothers of adults with mental retardation. *Family Relations, 50,* 154–163.

Hoyert, D. L., Kochaneck, K. D., & Murphy, S. L. (1999). *Deaths: Final data for 1997* (National Vital Statistics Reports, 47(19)). Hyattsville, MD: National Center for Health Statistics.

James, J., & Haley, W. (1995). Age and health bias in practicing clinical psychologists. *Psychology and Aging, 10,* 610–616.

Kraaij, V. W. de (2001). Negative life events and depressive symptoms in the elderly: A life-span perspective. *Aging and Mental Health, 5,* 84–91.

Laferriere, R. H., & Hamel-Bissell, B. P. (1994). Successful aging of oldest old women in the northeast kingdom of Vermont. *IMAGE: Journal of Nursing Scholarship, 26,* 319–323.

Lawton, M. P. (1975). The Philadelphia Geriatric Center Moral scale: A revision. *Journal of Gerontology, 30,* 85–94. Retrieved June 23, 2003, from http://www.qolid.org/public/pgc-ms/PGC_morale_scale.pdf

Luszcz, M. A., Bryan, J., & Kent, P. (1997). Predicting episodic memory performance of very old men and women: Contributions from age, depression, activity, cognitive ability and speed. *Psychology and Aging, 12,* 340–351.

Maruta, T., Colligan, R. C., Malinchoc, M., & Offord, K. P. (2000). Optimists vs. pessimists: Survival rate among medical patients over a 30 year period. *Mayo Clinic Proceedings, 75,* 140–143.

National Center for Health Statistics. (1998). *Health, United States, 1998.* Retrieved May 11, 2001, from http://www.cdc.gov/nchswww/data/hus98ncb.pdf

National Center for Health Statistics. (1999). *Health, United States, 1999.* Hyattsville, MD: Author.

Nelson, H. E., & Willison, J. (1991). National adult reading test (3rd ed.). Berkshire, England: NFER-Nelson.

Nordine, S., Monsch, A. U., & Murphy, C. (1995). Unawareness of smell loss in normal aging and Alzheimer's disease: Discrepancy between self reported and diagnosed smell sensitivity. *Journal of Gerontology: Psychological Sciences, 50,* 187–192.

North, C. S., Alpers, D. H., Thompson, S. J., & Spitznagel, E. L. (1996). Gastrointestinal symptoms and psychiatric disorders in the general population: Findings from the NIMH Epidemiologic Catchment Area Project. *Digestive Diseases and Sciences, 41,* 633–640.

Pinquart, M. (2001). Correlates of subjective health in older adults: A meta-analysis. *Psychology and Aging, 16,* 414–426.

Prenda, K. M., & Lachman, M. E. (2001). Planning for the future: A life management strategy for increasing control and life satisfaction in adulthood. *Psychology and Aging, 16,* 206–216.

Preville, M., Herbert, R., Boyer, R., & Bravo, G. (2001). Correlates of psychotropic drug use in the elderly compared to adults aged 18–64: Results from the Quebec Health Survey. *Aging & Mental Health, 5,* 216–224.

Scheibel, A. B. (1996). Structural and functional changes in the aging brain. In J. E. Birren & K. W. Schaie (Eds.), *Handbook of the psychology of aging* (4th ed., pp. 105–128). San Diego, CA: Academic Press.

Schroots, J. J. F. (1996). Theoretical developments in the psychology of aging. *The Gerontologist, 36*, 742–748.

Sheldon, K. M., & Kasser, T. (2001). Getting older? Getting better? Personal strivings and psychological maturity across the life span. *Developmental Psychology, 37*, 491–501.

Silver, J. M., Kramer, R., Greenwald, S., & Weissman, M. (2001). The association between head injuries and psychiatric disorders: Findings from the New Haven/NIMH Epidemiologic Catchment Area Study. *Brain Injury, 15*, 935–945.

Solomon, Z., & Ginzburg, K. (1998). War trauma and the aged: An Israeli perspective. In J. Lomranz (Ed.), *Handbook of aging and mental health: An integrative approach* (pp. 135–152). New York: Plenum Press.

Solomon, Z., & Ginzburg, K. (1999). Aging in the shadow of war. In A. Maercker, M. Schutzwohl, & Z. Solomon (Eds.), *Posttraumatic stress disorder: A lifespan developmental perspective* (pp. 137–153). Seattle, WA: Hogrefe & Huber.

Suitor, J. J., & Pillemer, K. (2000). When experience counts most: Effects of experiential similarity on men's and women's receipt of support during bereavement. *Social Networks, 22*, 299–312.

Tesch-Romer, C. (1997). Psychological effects of hearing aid use in older adults. *Journal of Gerontology: Psychological Sciences, 52*, 127–138.

Thomae, H. (1981). Expected unchangeability of life stress in old age: A contribution to a cognitive theory of aging. *Human Development, 24*, 229–239.

Thomae, H. (1990). Stress, satisfaction and competence: Findings from the Bonn Longitudinal Study on Aging. In M. Bergener & S. Finkel (Eds.), *Clinical and scientific psychogeriatrics: Vol. 1. The holistic approaches* (pp. 117–134). New York: Springer.

Tidball, K. (1990). Application of coping strategies developed by older deaf adults to the aging process. *American Annals of the Deaf, 135*, 33–40.

van Reekum, R., Cohen, T., & Wong, J. (2000). Can traumatic brain injury cause psychiatric disorders? *Journal of Neuropsychiatry and Clinical Neuroscience, 12*, 316–327.

Warr, P. (1998). Age, work and mental health. In K. W. Schaie & C. Schooler (Eds.), *The impact of work on older adults* (pp. 252–296). New York: Springer.

Wechsler, D. L. (1975). *Wechsler Adult Intelligence Scale* (3rd ed.). San Antonio, TX: Psychological Corporation.

Whitbourne, S. K. (1999). Physical changes. In J. C. Cavanaugh & S. K. Whitbourne (Eds.), *Gerontology: Interdisciplinary perspectives* (pp. 91–122). New York: Oxford University Press.

Wisocki, P. A., & Powers, P. A. (1997). Behavioral treatments for pain experienced by older adults. In D. I. Mostofsky & J. Lomranz (Eds.), *Handbook of pain and aging* (pp. 365–382). New York: Plenum Press.

Wood, V., Wylie, M. L., & Sheafor, B. (1969). An analysis of short self-report measure of life satisfaction: Correlation with rater judgments. *Journal of Gerontology, 24*, 465–469.

Wrosch, C., Heckhausen, J., & Lachman, M. E. (2000). Primary and secondary control strategies for managing health and financial stress across adulthood. *Psychology and Aging, 15*, 387–399.

II

HEALTH SYMPTOMS ASSOCIATED WITH FAMILY VIOLENCE

INTRODUCTION: HEALTH SYMPTOMS ASSOCIATED WITH FAMILY VIOLENCE

Screening for family violence is essential, but it is only the first step. Past or current abuse can manifest in a constellation of beliefs and behaviors that have a negative impact on health. In this section, five chapters describe common long-term manifestations of abuse. Each of these is described in detail, and the authors offer practical suggestions to help you work with clients who must overcome these problems. The authors recognize that it might not be you who provides these services. But knowing about them increases your ability to collaborate with those who do.

Chronic pain is the topic of the first chapter in this section. This is a common, and often costly, symptom of past abuse. This chapter describes the mechanisms by which abuse leads to chronic pain and describes treatment options available for pain patients.

Health risk behavior is another common symptom of abuse, and one that can lead to compromised health, revictimization, and premature death. Clinicians are often frustrated by the persistence of these behaviors. Chapter 10 offers some explanation for why these behaviors occur, and suggestions for how clinicians can help patients break the cycle of self-destructive behavior.

Childbearing is a common human experience, and abuse survivors often face additional challenges during this time. In chapter 11, the author guides clinicians through the childbearing year, highlighting some of the aspects of this experience that present challenges for many abuse survivors. It is one of the very few resources on this important topic.

Dissociation is a common symptom of trauma. What has not been appreciated, up until now, is how this symptom may manifest in health problems. Patients may ignore serious symptoms of illness because they are too frightened to seek care. Chapter 12 describes this phenomenon in compelling detail.

In the final chapter, traumatic brain injury is described. This is a common consequence for those who have been physically abused or assaulted. It often manifests as a psychiatric condition, such as depression. This chapter offers suggestions for assessment and intervention for a symptom that is frequently overlooked.

9

LINKS BETWEEN TRAUMATIC FAMILY VIOLENCE AND CHRONIC PAIN: BIOPSYCHOSOCIAL PATHWAYS AND TREATMENT IMPLICATIONS

MARY W. MEAGHER

Chronic pain is a common symptom among adult survivors of family violence. Indeed, it may be one of the most commonly occurring symptoms. This chapter explores the role of biopsychosocial factors in trauma and pain. It also offers a model for treating patients who have experienced family violence and now suffer from chronic pain.

Chronic pain patients have higher rates of sexual and physical abuse than normally occurs in the general population, suggesting that trauma plays a role in the development of chronic pain conditions (Drossman et al., 1990; Walker et al., 1999; Walker, Katon, Roy-Byrne, Jemelka, & Russo, 1993). Trauma during childhood or adulthood has also been shown to have a detrimental effect on emotional adjustment to chronic pain (Beckman et al., 1997; Geisser, Roth, Bachman, & Eckert, 1996; Spertus, Burns, Glenn, Lofland, & McCracken, 1999) and is associated with greater pain, distress, and disability (Amir et al., 1997; Linton, 1997; Scarinci, McDonald-Haile, Bradley, & Richter, 1994). The purpose of this chapter is to assist psychologists and other health care professionals in working with chronic pain patients who have experiences with traumatic family violence.

BACKGROUND AND THEORETICAL FOUNDATION

In this first section I provide essential background information and the theoretical rationale for integrating the treatment of chronic pain and traumatization. I begin by describing the various types of chronic pain syndromes and their psychosocial consequences. Next, I discuss the biopsychosocial model of chronic pain, gate control theory, and the biopsychosocial pathways linking trauma and chronic pain. I present an integrative model to guide the interventions outlined later in the chapter.

Chronic Pain Syndromes

Chronic pain refers to a variety of syndromes in which pain is present after the original injury has healed or in which pain is associated with a nonmalignant progressive disease (Ashbum & Staats, 1999; Gatchel & Turk, 1996). In progressive diseases, such as rheumatoid arthritis, pain is due to the persistent stimulation of nociceptors in areas of ongoing inflammation and tissue damage. In other cases, pain is due to injury-induced sensitization of pain transmission pathways in the peripheral and central nervous system (e.g., Woolf & Mannion, 1999). Other chronic pain syndromes are triggered by autoimmunity and infectious agents that sensitize pain pathways (Watkins & Maier, 2000). Finally, many patients present without any known initiating injury, infection, or progressive disease. Indeed, relatively little is known about the pathophysiology of many chronic pain syndromes (Ashbum & Staats, 1999; Gatchel & Turk, 1996). Consequently, clinicians often lack the laboratory tests or objective clinical criteria to diagnose many chronic pain syndromes, including chronic low back pain, neuropathic and myofascial pain, fibromyalgia, headache, and central pain syndromes.

Chronic pain patients frequently experience significant psychological distress and functional disability, including depression, anxiety, substance abuse, sleep disturbance, and fatigue, resulting in decreased physical, social, and occupational functioning (Turk, 1996). A vicious cycle occurs by which pain produces stress and tension, which in turn cause more pain. Over time, many patients become emotionally drained and demoralized when their pain continues despite multiple treatments. Skeptical about obtaining pain relief, they do not adhere to their treatment regimen and are reluctant to collaborate with health care providers. As pain increasingly dominates their life, they become physically inactive and socially disengaged. This downward spiral can become infectious, leading to frustration and negative reactions on the part of families, friends, health care providers, and employers.

Biomedical and Biopsychosocial Models of Chronic Pain

Interventions used to manage chronic pain are derived from the basic assumptions regarding factors that cause and maintain disease (Turk, 1996). The biomedical model focuses on pathophysiology and objective biological manifestations of chronic pain. From this perspective, pain is caused and maintained by biological processes that can be objectively measured; accordingly, treatment involves medical or surgical approaches to correct the biological dysfunction. Although recent advances in biomedical research have increased our understanding of pain mechanisms, biological factors alone do not provide a complete account of chronic pain. Observable pathophysiology is often poorly correlated with the severity of pain, distress, and disability (Waddell, 1987). For example, patients with the same level of objective physical pathology receiving back surgery respond very differently (North, Campbell, & James, 1991). One patient experiences pain relief, while the other continues to experience severe pain.

To understand the variability inherent in chronic pain, medical and mental health professionals need a biopsychosocial model that considers the complex reciprocal interactions between biological, psychological, and social factors that shape the patient's experience and responses to pain (Turk, 1996). This model acknowledges that the patient's subjective experience of pain, and its social consequences, play an important role in determining the severity and course of chronic pain. For example, the psychological experience of stress influences the appraisal or perception of pain sensations and affects biological processes (e.g., dysregulation of the hypothalamic–pituitary–adrenal axis, sympathetic outflow, immune activation, and descending modulatory pathways) that contribute to the onset, modulation, and maintenance of chronic pain.

Gate control theory provided the first integrative model that addressed the role of both psychological and physiological factors in pain (Melzack & Wall, 1965). Although many of the physiological details of this model have required revision, the general theoretical concepts have held up, especially its capacity to explain the complex interactions of psychological and biological factors in determining pain perception. According to this theory, pain signals are normally carried by sensory fibers from the site of injury to neurons in the spinal cord and from there to the brain (see Figure 9.1, left side). Within the spinal cord, an area called the *dorsal horn* acts as a "gate" that can be opened or closed. When the gate is open, signals are transmitted to the brain, where they are experienced as pain sensation if they are sufficiently intense. When the gate is closed, the magnitude of the incoming signal is inhibited, and pain sensation is reduced. Most important for the present purposes is the dynamic role that the brain plays in pain processing and perception. The brain sends signals down into the spinal cord that

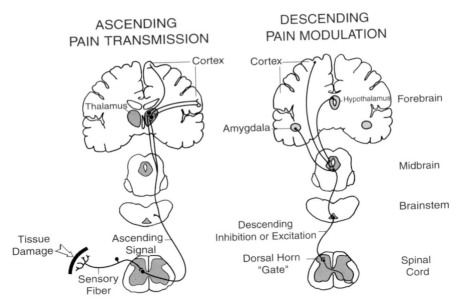

ASCENDING
PAIN TRANSMISSION

DESCENDING
PAIN MODULATION

Cortex

Cortex

Thalamus

Hypothalamus Forebrain

Amygdala

Midbrain

Brainstem

Descending
Inhibition or Excitation

Tissue
Damage

Ascending
Signal

Dorsal Horn
"Gate"

Spinal
Cord

Sensory
Fiber

Figure 9.1. The ascending pain transmission pathway (left side of figure) and the descending pain modulatory pathway (right side of figure). The ascending pain transmission pathway carries pain signals from the periphery through the spinal cord to the brain. The arrow at the lower left represents a painful stimulus that activates a sensory fiber. This sensory fiber terminates in the dorsal horn of the spinal cord, where it relays the pain signal to a pain transmission neuron, which in turn carries the signal to the brain. The descending pain modulatory pathway regulates pain transmission in the spinal cord. The pathway is influenced by projections from forebrain structures involved in affect regulation. In the spinal cord, this descending pathway controls a gating mechanism (dorsal horn) that can either facilitate or inhibit the incoming pain signal. From *Animal Research and Human Health: Advancing Human Welfare Through Behavioral Science* (pp. 230, 234), by M. E. Carroll and J. B. Overmier (Eds.), 2001, Washington, DC: American Psychological Association. Copyright 2001 by American Psychological Association. Adapted with permission.

affect this gating mechanism (see Figure 9.1, right side). Through these descending neural pathways, the brain can either amplify or inhibit the transmission of incoming signals, determining the intensity of pain that is experienced. For example, an anxious person will experience more intense pain, because the brain opens the gate and amplifies pain processing to promote hypervigilance in potentially dangerous situations. In contrast, the brain can send an inhibitory signal that closes the gate during positive emotions. This descending modulatory pathway provides one mechanism whereby emotions and thoughts can influence pain intensity (Fields, 2000). In addition, emotion may influence pain at the level of the brain through activation of neural structures shared by emotion and pain circuits (Rhudy & Meagher, 2001).

BIOPSYCHOSOCIAL PATHWAYS LINKING TRAUMA AND CHRONIC PAIN

When chronic pain occurs in the context of family violence, it is important to understand the bidirectional relationships that exist between biological, psychological, and social processes mediating chronic pain and trauma. Although many of the psychosocial problems associated with chronic pain (e.g., stress, depression) are reactive and attributable to the stress of living with chronic pain, heightened levels of stress can lead to alterations in biological processes, which in turn exacerbate pain. In situations of current family violence, the stress of living with abuse is likely to intensify this vicious cycle. Below I review the biopsychosocial pathways by which family violence may contribute to chronic pain.

Changes Initiated by Physical Injury

One obvious biological pathway involves the neuropathic changes initiated by physical injury itself (e.g., Woolf & Mannion, 1999). For many chronic pain syndromes, a tissue-damaging event sensitizes the pain transmission pathway, resulting in a "pain memory" that persists long after the original injury has healed. From this perspective, damage to the genitals and rectum during childhood sexual abuse could play an etiological role in chronic pelvic and gastrointestinal pain syndromes. Support for this view comes from clinical studies linking sexual abuse to chronic pelvic and gastrointestinal pain (e.g., Drossman et al., 1990; Lampe et al., 2000; Leserman et al., 1996; Scarinci et al., 1994; Walker et al., 1999; Walker et al., 1993; Walling et al., 1994). Additional studies have found a relationship between abuse and other forms of chronic pain, such as headache and back pain (Amir et al., 1997; Linton, 1997; Spertus et al., 1999; Walling et al., 1994). Although previous studies have focused on childhood trauma, sexual and physical abuse during adulthood also increase vulnerability to chronic pain and other adverse health outcomes (Leserman et al., 1996; Spertus et al., 1999).

It is unclear whether the relationship between abuse and chronic pain reflects injury-induced changes in pain transmission pathways, or dysregulation of pain modulatory systems due to psychological trauma, or both. Animal studies indicate that exposure to noxious stimuli early in development can trigger the neuroanatomical reorganization of pain pathways and cause hyperexcitability in peripheral and central neurons that persists into adulthood (e.g., Ruda et al., 2000). Other evidence suggests that exposure to aversive stimuli during adulthood can sensitize the pain circuits and dysregulate descending modulatory systems that normally inhibit incoming pain signals (Fields, 2000; Woolf & Mannion, 1999). These modulatory systems become dysregulated, in part, because limbic and brain stem structures that contribute to both pain and affect modulation are sensitized by exposure to traumatic events (Rhudy & Meagher, 2001; Rosen & Schulkin, 1998). These findings suggest that injury and associated stress alter pain transmission and modulatory pathways, contributing to the etiology and maintenance of chronic pain.

Chronic Psychological Stress

Physical abuse occurs within a larger context of emotional abuse, including threats, intimidation, coercion, humiliation, and social isolation. Chronic psychological stress contributes to the development of depression, anxiety, and affect dysregulation, resulting in higher levels of pain-related emotional distress, lower levels of perceived control, and an impaired ability to cope with pain and daily hassles (Cohen & Rodriguez, 1996; Lautenbacher, Spernal, Schreiber, & Krieg, 1999; Linton, 1997). At a physiological level, chronic psychosocial stress results in prolonged exposure to high levels of stress hormones that can dysregulate neural, immune, endocrine, and other organ systems, predisposing the individual to a range of stress-related disorders, including chronic pain (Ehlert, Gaab, & Heinrichs, 2001; McEwen, 2000; Meaney, 2001; Stephan, Helfritz, Pabst, & von Horsten, 2002; van der Kolk et al., 1996).

It is important to note that posttraumatic stress disorder (PTSD) and chronic pain share common psychological and neural mechanisms that may make them mutually maintaining conditions (Rosen & Schulkin, 1998; Sharp & Harvey, 2001). Both conditions are commonly observed after traumatic events and are associated with affect dysregulation caused by stress-induced changes in limbic and cortical circuits implicated in emotion and pain modulation. Several mechanisms contribute to the mutual maintenance of these disorders, including: (a) hypervigilance and anxiety, (b) attentional and reasoning biases, (c) anxiety sensitivity and catastrophizing, (d) sensitization, (e) conditioned fears, (f) avoidance, (g) depression and reduced activity, and (h) cognitive demands that interfere with adaptive coping. Understanding the mechanisms by which mutual maintenance occurs may be useful in guiding interventions designed to enhance affect regulation.

Integrative Model

An integrative model (depicted in Figure 9.2) can be used to understand how PTSD and chronic pain develop from normal fear and pain responses (Foa & Rothbaum, 1998; Rosen & Schulkin, 1998; van der Kolk et al., 1996). Fear responses are normally short lived and decline once the individual begins to cope with the threatening event. Likewise, incoming pain

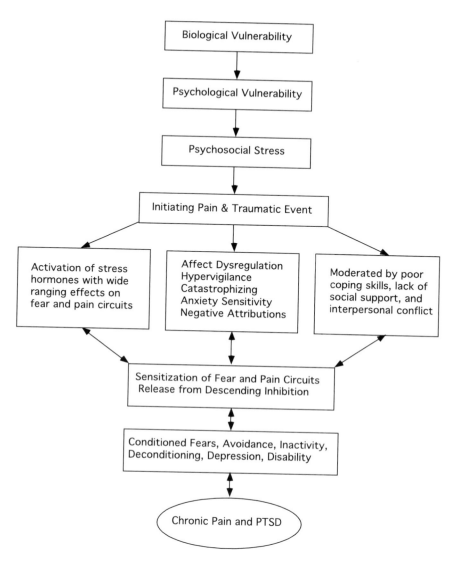

Figure 9.2. An integrative model of the biopsychosocial pathways through which traumatic family violence may contribute to the development and exacerbation of chronic pain. PTSD = posttraumatic stress disorder.

signals are normally gated by descending inhibitory systems when pain is manageable. However, after psychosocial stress the neural structures shared by fear and pain circuits are overactivated, causing a cascade of cognitive, behavioral, and neurobiological changes that contribute to the development of pathological anxiety and chronic pain. With repeated activation, reduced thresholds and hyperexcitability can develop through a sensitization process.

This hyperexcitability manifests itself behaviorally as hypervigilance, increased responsiveness to unconditioned and conditioned aversive stimuli, increased associative and avoidance conditioning, and reduced activity (Rosen & Schulkin, 1998; Sharp & Harvey, 2001).

Exaggerated responses to pain- and trauma-related stimuli develop through classical conditioning (Shors, Weiss, & Thompson, 1992) as well as through unconditioned sensitization of fear and pain responses (Rhudy & Meagher, 2001). Operant conditioning mechanisms subsequently contribute to the maintenance of anxiety and pain behaviors (Foa & Rothbaum, 1998; Gatchel & Turk, 1996). The individual learns to reduce anxiety through avoidance or escape from unconditioned and conditioned aversive stimuli by means of the process of negative reinforcement, whereas observable pain behaviors may be maintained through contingent social reinforcement (solicitous responses) by means of the process of positive reinforcement. Over time, the activation of fear and pain behaviors can be triggered by cues outside of conscious awareness, leading to a feeling of loss of control. In addition, hypervigilance and attentional and reasoning biases lead the patient to perceive and respond to stimuli as threatening. These cognitive demands can become so severe that they impair social and occupational functioning.

Susceptibility to PTSD and chronic pain is partly explained by the severity of trauma and physical pathology (Resnick, Kilpatrick, Dansky, Saunders, & Best, 1993; Waddell, 1987). However, three vulnerability factors are likely to contribute (Foy, Resnick, Sipprelle, & Carroll, 1987; Schofferman, Anderson, Hinds, Smith, & White, 1992): (a) genetic predispositions, (b) childhood neglect and trauma, and (c) psychosocial stress and trauma throughout the life span. A diathesis–stress model can be used to understand the interaction between these factors. People who develop PTSD and chronic pain may possess a genetic vulnerability to overreact to stress and pain (True et al., 1993). They may also possess psychological vulnerabilities based on early experiences with unpredictable or uncontrollable aversive events (Foy et al., 1987; Schofferman et al., 1992). Finally, intrapersonal and interpersonal factors, such as coping skills and social support, protect one from the effects of stress and therefore from developing PTSD and chronic pain disorders (Bradley, 1996; Vernberg, La Greca, Silverman, & Prinstein, 1996).

Posttraumatic stress disorder and chronic pain appear to develop from normal fear and pain responses when psychosocial stress sensitizes fear and pain circuits. If trauma or physical pathology occurs in a person who has been subjected to past or present family violence, the consequent sensitization of fear and pain circuits increases the likelihood that he or she will develop PTSD and chronic pain. As a corollary, individuals with adequate coping skills and social support should have reduced activation of fear and pain circuits and increased descending inhibitory control over incoming pain signals. Prior experiences with control over aversive stimuli should further reduce sensitization. From this perspective, psychological interventions that involve coping skills training, social support, and exposure therapies should enhance perceived control and reduce stress while desensitizing fear and pain circuits.

A GUIDE TO INTEGRATING CHRONIC PAIN AND PTSD TREATMENT

In this section I describe how to integrate cognitive–behavioral therapy (CBT) for traumatization and chronic pain. I begin by describing the integral role that psychologists and other mental health providers play in interdisciplinary pain management. Next, I discuss how to tailor the psychological assessment and intervention process for chronic pain patients who are victims of traumatic family violence. I also describe how psychologists can work with other health care providers to enhance detection and treatment.

Interdisciplinary Pain Management

Interdisciplinary approaches to pain management, which address all the dimensions of the patient's condition, have been shown to improve functioning in chronic pain patients (Turk, 1995). Improvements are observed across a range of measures, including pain reduction, reduction of opioid medication, activity increase, return to work, reduction in health care utilization, and closure of disability cases. These improvements result in substantial cost savings from the standpoint of patients, third-party payers, claims adjusters, and society.

Most interdisciplinary treatment teams involve a physician, a psychologist, a physical therapist, an occupational therapist, a nurse, and a pharmacist—all with expertise in pain management (Ashbum & Staats, 1999; Turk, 1995). Although each team member makes a unique contribution to patient care, coordination of care is essential for effective treatment. After an initial screening, all members of the team meet to develop a treatment plan tailored to the individual needs of the patient. In collaboration with the patient, the team identifies realistic and measurable treatment goals. Treatment goals may include pain reduction, identification and modification of dysfunctional attitudes and attributions, development of active coping skills, improved mood and sleep, increased physical and social functioning, reduction in opioid medication, improved treatment adherence, and return to work.

Treatment plans can range from brief patient education and pharmacological management to more extensive rehabilitation programs involving multiple treatment modalities. For example, the physician may use nerve blocks to reduce pain to increase adherence to physical therapy with the goal of improving physical conditioning. At the same time, the physical therapist and psychologist can work together to reduce pain-related fear-avoidance beliefs and behaviors, with physical therapy as a venue for in vivo exposure therapy. This is helpful for patients who avoid physical activity and experience deconditioning because of fears of reinjury. The psychologist also addresses problems with coping, depression, substance abuse, motivation, treatment adherence, sleep disturbance, interpersonal problems, response of significant others, and secondary gain. Psychological management must be coordinated with the physician, pharmacist, and nurse, who monitor the patient's response to antidepressant, sleep, muscle tension, and analgesic medications.

In most interdisciplinary treatment models, CBT is used to treat a variety of chronic pain syndromes (Bradley, 1996; Turk, Meichenbaum, Genest, 1983). The goal is to modify the patient's understanding of pain and his or her negative expectancies and attributions and to develop more adaptive cognitive and behavioral coping strategies. When chronic pain occurs against a backdrop of family violence and trauma, the level of psychological distress and functional disability is likely to be even greater and to require treatment components that are not normally included in standard CBT. These patients are more likely to suffer from severe depression, PTSD, substance abuse, and personality disorders, which require a combination of CBT, operant, prolonged exposure, relapse prevention, interpersonal, and dialectical treatment components. In other cases, victims of family violence react with relatively normal emotional reactions (e.g., anger, fear, sadness). Although they do not meet diagnostic criteria, these patients are at risk for developing adjustment problems. For these patients, standard CBT for chronic pain and exposure therapy for trauma can be used to prevent more severe dysfunction (Bradley, 1996; Foa & Rothbaum, 1998).

INTEGRATING COGNITIVE–BEHAVIORAL THERAPY FOR CHRONIC PAIN AND TRAUMATIZATION

Much has been written on how to manage chronic pain with CBT, but the treatment of co-occurring traumatization has received little attention. In the sections that follow, I describe how to tailor the psychological management of chronic pain in victims of traumatic family violence focusing on PTSD. Several practical issues need to be addressed when integrating treatment. These issues include establishing the rationale for psychological intervention, conducting pretreatment screening and assessment for traumatic family violence and chronic pain, implementing an individualized treatment plan to help patients cope with their pain and trauma, and developing a plan to maintain these gains after treatment has ended.

Therapeutic Alliance and Rationale

During the initial contact, the psychologist explains the rationale for psychological intervention and begins to establish a therapeutic alliance. In many cases, patients negatively interpret the psychological referral as evidence that their provider views their pain as "all in their head." It is important for a psychologist to let the patient know that he or she thinks that the patient's pain is real but that it cannot be eliminated by current medical or surgical treatments. Then the psychologist should explain that the goal of interdisciplinary pain management is to control pain so that the patient can function better and should clarify that psychologists are involved in pain management because they can help patients learn skills to control and decrease their pain and the stress it creates. During this discussion, the psychologist must be careful to depathologize the patient's difficulties in coping by discussing the vicious cycle of pain and stress. This can be addressed by describing how chronic pain can lead to the stressors that the patient reports (e.g., anger, depression, isolation), which in turn can increase pain. The psychologist should then describe how other psychosocial stressors, including family violence, can feed into this cycle and further amplify the patient's level of pain and stress.

With the understanding that many patients come to psychological treatment after a series of invalidating experiences, the following guidelines are recommended to develop a working alliance (Foa & Rothbaum, 1998):

1. Adopt an empathic and nonjudgmental stance when patients discuss their experiences with chronic pain and trauma.
2. Demonstrate expertise and confidence to enhance treatment acceptance, trust, and safety.
3. Acknowledge the patient's strengths and his or her courage to seek treatment.
4. Normalize the patient's response to family violence and chronic pain, which communicates that you do not view the patient as weak, pathological, or malingering.

Pretreatment Assessment

Before a treatment plan can be developed, a thorough pretreatment assessment of the patient's chronic pain and abuse history should be conducted. Pretreatment evaluation sessions are needed to guide treatment and to screen for other conditions (e.g., substance dependence, suicidal ideation) that need to be addressed before they can benefit from treatment. Pretreatment assessment also provides baseline measures of target behaviors to evaluate the patient's response to treatment.

Because each patient's needs are unique, the psychologist must use his or her clinical judgment to decide how to sequence the assessment process. A battered woman presenting in an emergency room with a broken arm and a history of back pain has obviously different needs than a woman presenting in a primary care setting with chronic pelvic pain and a sexual abuse history. In the former case, family violence should be the initial focus of assessment; in the latter case, the assessment process should begin with the presenting pain problem, but screening for family violence should occur later in the session (Bradley, Haile, & Jaworski, 1992).

Identification and Assessment of Family Violence and Trauma

Identification of sexual and physical abuse can be difficult, because victims frequently deny or minimize their abuse out of fear or shame. Screening questions that inquire about concrete behavioral indicators of violence (e.g., punching, choking, forced sexual contact, threats to harm or kill) are more likely to identify abused patients than are questions with general labels (e.g., violence, physical abuse, rape, psychological abuse; Dutton, Haywood, & El-Bayoumi, 1997; Gondolf, 1998). Screening should be followed by an abuse history and administration of abuse and lethality inventories to determine the nature, extent, duration, and risks of abuse (Gondolf, 1998). In cases of ongoing family violence, the first priority is to assess the patient's safety and risks to children and other family members. After present or potential danger has been evaluated, the level of psychological distress should be assessed so one can determine whether more extensive psychological evaluation is required. Depression, anxiety, dissociation, poor self-image, self-blame, sexual dysfunction, and suppressed anger are common responses to family violence (Gondolf, 1998). In many cases, these symptoms do not precede the abuse history and are related to PTSD. Research indicates that PTSD affects 45% to 55% of women in battered women programs and 75% of women in acute crisis centers (Gondolf, 1998). Patients with PTSD exhibit a range of avoidance, intrusive re-experiencing, and arousal symptoms that can be mistaken for other disorders. Thus, diagnoses of personality disorders and other conditions should not be made unless PTSD has been ruled out.

A PTSD diagnosis involves several assessment methods (Foa & Rothbaum, 1998). Clinical interviews are used to collect information regarding abuse, preabuse adjustment, and stressful events prior to abuse as well as the patient's reactions to the abuse. When discussing the abuse itself, the patient should be allowed to tell his or her story, but the psychologists should provide occasional empathic and reassuring comments. For some patients, the Assault Information and History Interview (Foa & Rothbaum, 1998) and other structured interviews can be used to guide the clinical interview. A number of standardized clinician-administered and self-report measures of PTSD are also available (e.g., Clinician-Administered PTSD Scale, PTSD Symptoms Severity Scale, PTSD Diagnostic Scale, and the Impact of Events Scale (Foa, Riggs, Dancu, & Rothbaum, 1993; Horowitz, Wilner, & Alvarez, 1979). Self-monitoring can also be used to record target behaviors and to evaluate the relationship between pain and PTSD symptoms.

Chronic Pain Assessment

Pretreatment assessment of chronic pain should evaluate (a) the location, intensity, and quality of the pain; (b) factors that increase or decrease pain; (c) the patient's family-, social-, and work-related activities to identify adaptive and maladaptive behaviors; (d) cognitive factors, including beliefs, irrational thoughts, and negative expectancies; (e) mood and affective responses that alter pain; and (f) the patient's pain history, treatment history, and current treatments (Bradley et al., 1992; Kerns & Jacob, 1992; Turk et al., 1983; Turk & Melzack, 1992). Prepain adjustment should also be evaluated to determine prior experiences in coping with pain and stress; problem-solving skills; and family, social, occupational, and legal system functioning.

Several assessment methods can be used to understand the nature of the patient's pain and how it affects his or her life. A pain diary can be helpful in identifying thoughts, behaviors, moods, and interpersonal and environmental factors that influence pain as well as the strategies that the patient uses to cope with pain (Turk et al., 1983). Self-monitoring not only increases the patient's awareness of the psychological and situational determinants of pain, but it also can be used throughout treatment to evaluate progress. To determine the relationship between pain and PTSD symptoms, practitioners should design self-monitoring sheets to record cues and target behaviors associated with each condition. Standardized measures, such as the McGill Pain Questionnaire (Melzack & Katz, 1992) and the Multidimensional Pain Inventory (Kerns & Jacob, 1992), can provide information regarding the nature of the pain and the psychosocial context, respectively. The Minnesota Multiphasic Personality Inventory and the Millon Behavioral Health Inventory (Millon, Green, & Meagher, 1982; Butcher, Dahlstrom, Graham, Tellegen, & Kaemmer, 1989) are the most commonly used (Bradley et al., 1992) measures to evaluate psychological status. Additional measures of depression, anxiety, marital satisfaction, substance use, and coping style can also be used. The patient's motivation for treatment and perceived self-efficacy should be evaluated to match the treatment components to the patient's stage of change (Gatchel & Turk, 1996). If appropriate, significant others can be interviewed separately or in a partner–patient interview to understand (a) how the family system is affected by pain and (b) the influence of family system on pain (Bradley, 1996; Turk et al., 1983).

In parallel with psychological assessment, the patient should be referred for a physical examination to evaluate the presenting pain complaint and to document any current or past injuries. This should include injuries sustained during direct physical or sexual assault as well as injuries sustained during attempts at escape, avoidance, retaliation, or as the primary aggressor. If current or recent injuries are identified, the physician should determine the stage or stages of healing and whether they are related to the chronic pain and trauma syndrome. It is also important to document medical problems that are not directly related to injury or chronic pain, because victims of family violence experience a wide range of health problems.

The initial evaluation usually takes two to three sessions, but the process of assessment continues throughout treatment to determine response to treatment and when to terminate treatment. The information gathered during the assessment phase should be used to develop a set of treatment goals in collaboration with the patient and the interdisciplinary team.

Individualized Treatment Planning

If the psychologist concludes that the patient could benefit from some form of psychological treatment, then he or she needs to prioritize the patient's problems to decide which treatment components to begin with (Foa & Rothbaum, 1998; Turk et al., 1983). For many patients, education, relaxation training, and prolonged exposure therapy will be effective, whereas others will require additional components to address dysfunctional thoughts and extreme stress (e.g., cognitive restructuring and stress inoculation training). Sequencing of intervention components should be prioritized in light of the patient's current level of pain, traumatization, and coping skills.

Cognitive–behavioral therapy for chronic pain involves four components: (a) education, (b) skill acquisition and rehearsal, (c) cognitive and behavioral rehearsal, and (d) generalization and maintenance (Bradley, 1996; Turk et al., 1983). Cognitive–behavioral therapy for trauma focuses on prolonged-exposure techniques and selected components of stress inoculation therapy (Foa & Rothbaum, 1998). Integrative CBT will usually involve 20 to 30 weekly sessions, but some patients respond in fewer sessions, whereas others take longer. Patients who do not show substantial improvement after 15 sessions are unlikely to benefit from additional CBT alone. In such cases, the treatment plan needs to be re-evaluated and other components (e.g., motivational enhancement, interpersonal, or couple therapy) considered.

Education

The goal of education is to help the patient understand the rationale for psychological intervention, to foster a therapeutic alliance, and to develop a shared conceptualization of pain (Turk et al., 1983). In cases of family violence, the initial education phase addresses how abuse and its psychosocial consequences contribute to chronic pain. In the absence of education, patients often maintain dualistic views of pain and trauma, tending to view pain as physical and trauma as psychological. Until the patient and psychologist develop a shared conceptualization that explains the links between chronic pain and trauma, they are likely to work at cross-purposes.

The biopsychosocial model of chronic pain and trauma and the gate control theory described earlier should be discussed (Turk et al., 1983). During this discussion, patients are asked to identify thoughts, emotions, and events that influence their pain and alter the gating of pain signals. Likewise, they should be asked to identify the psychological and environmental factors that elicit PTSD symptoms. Patients frequently report that negative emotions and thoughts exacerbate both conditions, whereas pleasant emotions, perceived control, and absorption in activities reduce them. They are also asked to describe ways in which they can manage their pain and stress reactions as well as factors that contribute to a perceived loss of control and nonadherence to treatment. Through this discussion, patients learn about the impact on their pain and trauma syndromes of stress and cognitive appraisal. They also learn that they can control their reactions to pain and even the intensity of their pain. The role of family violence and significant others who inadvertently reinforce pain behaviors should be addressed, as should the impact of the patient's pain on social and occupational functioning. Next, patients are told how the components of CBT are designed to enhance their control over pain and stress. Patients are told that they will learn to control their pain and stress by changing the emotions and thoughts that modulate their pain and PTSD symptoms.

Skill Acquisition and Rehearsal

After the education phase, treatment focuses on skill acquisition and rehearsal (Bradley, 1996; Foa & Rothbaum, 1998; Turk et al., 1983). Patients learn new skills through behavioral rehearsal in session and homework assignments. Behavioral rehearsal involves instruction in a coping skill, patient rehearsal, and therapist feedback. Before and after rehearsal, the patient assesses his or her level of pain and stress to measure progress. The therapist provides feedback on the patient's performance along with suggestions on how to use the coping skill more effectively. After a skill has been practiced in session or as a homework assignment, patients are asked to identify high-risk situations that might interfere with practicing the skill or with using it in their everyday lives. Then they are asked to identify ways to cope with these high-risk situations. Because most patients experience some symptom relief and perceived control with relaxation and breathing retraining, these are usually the first skills to be taught. Cognitive coping skills such as pleasant imagery and distraction are also readily mastered. For some patients, cognitive restructuring can be used to identify and correct irrational fears, catastrophizing, attentional and attributional biases, and other maladaptive thoughts as well as to reinforce positive self-efficacy beliefs and other adaptive thoughts. Behavioral skills such as setting realistic activity goals, activity–rest cycling, and communication skills to manage family conflicts are also taught.

To address trauma and fears of reinjury, one uses imaginal and *in vivo* exposure interventions to reduce sensitization, conditioned fears, and cognitive and behavioral avoidance. For these interventions to be effective, the patient must become physiologically aroused during the initial exposure, and the session must be long enough to allow the level of arousal to decline during the session and across repeated sessions (Foa & Rothbaum, 1998). Prolonged exposure appears to facilitate the restructuring of emotional schema at both an emotional and cognitive level, whereas short exposure sessions may result in resensitization if there is inadequate time for dissipating elicited arousal and recasting of the emotional memory. Prolonged-exposure therapies should reduce sensitization of fear and pain circuits, thereby decreasing attentional biases, hypervigilance, anxiety sensitivity, conditioned fear, and avoidance behavior.

As patients become desensitized and acquire new coping skills, they develop more adaptive beliefs and expectancies about pain and stress and increased self-efficacy. Over time, patients learn to become active problem-solvers as they practice their newly acquired coping skills and progressively increase their activity levels. Throughout treatment, the psychologist discourages discussions that focus on the patient's pain or negative affect. If appropriate, supportive family members can be taught to reinforce adaptive thoughts and behaviors while ignoring pain behaviors and discussions that focus on pain and traumatic rumination (Bradley, 1996; Foa & Rothbaum, 1998).

Generalization and Maintenance

The goal of the generalization and maintenance phase is to help patients maintain their skills after treatment and thus prevent relapse (Bradley, 1996; Gatchel & Turk, 1996). Patients are asked to identify potential high-risk situations that might occur after therapy by examining situational, interpersonal, and intrapersonal factors surrounding past relapses. They then explore ways to cope with these high-risk situations so that they continue to use their coping skills and avoid increases in pain and stress after treatment. First, they learn how to identify the cues that lead to relapse and to immediately use coping skills, such as relaxation, to prevent escalation. Next, they are taught to evaluate the situational factors that contributed to the lapse or relapse. Finally, they identify coping strategies that can be implemented when these high-risk situations occur in the future. Role playing how he or she might cope with the high-risk situation can increase the patient's skill level and self-efficacy, thereby reducing the likelihood of future relapse. It is important to emphasize that increases in pain and trauma symptoms be viewed not as failures but as cues to use their coping skills and to develop more realistic goals, behavioral strategies, or rewards for coping. Again, supportive family members should be involved in relapse prevention training to enhance maintenance. Monthly phone calls can be scheduled three to six months after treatment to facilitate maintenance of coping skills.

Working With Other Health Care Professionals

Victims of family violence and chronic pain are more likely to present in primary care and emergency rooms than in mental health settings. To facilitate the detection and treatment of these patients, psychologists need to educate other health care providers about the biopsychosocial model linking chronic pain and family violence. When providers understand this model, they are more likely to support routine screening, referral for psychological services, interdisciplinary pain management, and collaborative treatment (Turk et al., 1983).

A number of barriers interfere with routine screening for family violence in chronic pain patients (Dutton et al., 1997). Providers often have limited knowledge regarding the prevalence and demographics of family violence. For example, they may assume that patients of higher socioeconomic status, elderly patients, or religious patients are less likely to be victims of family violence. Many providers feel that they lack the time and training to effectively screen for violence and pain. Moreover, they are often uncertain about how to use the screening information to guide referral and treatment. Although many providers fear that patients will be offended when they inquire about abuse, most patients report feeling comfortable discussing these issues and consider it relevant to their medical care (Friedman, Samet, Roberts, & Hans, 1992). Another barrier is the frustration that providers experience when pain patients, receiving multiple referrals for testing and specialty care, return reporting more stress and pain than before. They can become even more frustrated when victims of abuse do not follow advice to leave the abusive situation, especially in situations of extreme violence or where children are at risk.

Health psychologists serving in consultation and liaison positions can play an important role in overcoming these barriers. They can work with other providers to implement routine screening and referral programs for violence and chronic pain. Providers should be informed that family violence occurs across all socioeconomic levels and across all cultural, religious, professional, age, and gender groups. Screening protocols should follow the guidelines described above to identify patients at risk of severe physical or sexual abuse before violence escalates. To increase the use of screening, one should provide clear guidelines and contact information for referral, assessment, and treatment. Although screening is advised, it is important to recognize that charting and disclosure of this information can have unintended consequences. For example, health insurance coverage could be denied because of a pre-existing condition (Walker et al., 1999). Providers should understand the sensitive nature of sexual and physical abuse and be careful to protect patient confidentiality (see also chap. 1, this volume).

Health psychologists can help other providers establish collaborative relationships with patients to foster safety and active coping while helping the provider to understand and manage their reactions to these challenging patients. Primary care providers are in a unique position to manage many of the adverse emotional and physical consequences of family violence and chronic pain. These patients are likely to benefit from a stable therapeutic alliance with a supportive physician who responds to their emotional and physical problems with empathy, acceptance, and respect. A strong alliance can help providers promote lifestyle changes that reduce health risk behaviors to improve the patient's emotional and physical health.

Finally, psychologists working with victims of family violence in mental health settings should screen for chronic pain and other health problems. Most psychologists can use relaxation training, prolonged exposure, cognitive restructuring, and other CBT interventions to help these patients manage their pain and PTSD and reduce health risk behaviors. Rather than work in isolation, psychologists should coordinate care with the patient's physician and other providers. They can also refer patients for interdisciplinary pain management or other specialty care for health risk behaviors (e.g., smoking, alcohol abuse, obesity) that may fall outside their expertise.

CONCLUSION

Traumatic family violence is linked to the development and exacerbation of chronic pain. Deficits in affect regulation following trauma and chronic pain appear to be related to stress-induced sensitization of neural structures shared by fear and pain circuits. Patients experience wide-ranging and intense emotions that interfere with their ability to focus on activities of daily living and reduce their ability to inhibit behaviors triggered by feelings of fear, anger, and depression. Over time, the threshold for eliciting negative affect and pain is lowered. As patients lose their ability to modulate emotion and pain, they exhibit high levels of negative affect and functional disability. The intensification and focus on negative affect can amplify incoming pain signals, creating a vicious cycle. Sensitization, classical and operant conditioning, and cognitive processes contribute to the development and maintenance of exaggerated responses to pain- and trauma-related stimuli.

The psychological management of co-occurring chronic pain and traumatization is guided by this biopsychosocial perspective and focuses on coping skills training and exposure therapies designed to enhance perceived control and affect regulation while desensitizing fear and pain circuits. Although future research is needed to evaluate the effectiveness of integrating CBT for chronic pain and PTSD, integrative treatment should improve outcome because these conditions appear to be mutually maintaining (Sharp & Harvey, 2001). Integrative CBT should ideally occur within the context of interdisciplinary pain management that addresses the biological and psychosocial dimensions of chronic pain (Turk, 1995, 1996). To increase detection and treatment of family violence in chronic pain patients, we recommend that providers practice routine screening in primary care and emergency room settings.

REFERENCES

Amir, M., Kaplan, Z., Neumann, L., Sharabani, R., Shani, N., & Buskila, D. (1997). Posttraumatic stress disorder tenderness and fibromyalgia. *Journal of Psychosomatic Research, 42*, 607–613.

Ashbum, M. A., & Staats, P. S. (1999). Management of chronic pain. *The Lancet, 353*, 1865–1869.

Beckman, J. C., Crawford, A. L., Feldman, M. E., Kirby, A. C., Hertzberg, M. A., Davidson, J. R. T., & Moore, S. D. (1997). Chronic posttraumatic stress disorder and chronic pain in Vietnam combat veterans. *Journal of Psychosomatic Research, 43*, 379–389.

Bradley, L. A. (1996). Cognitive–behavioral therapy for chronic pain. In R. J. Gatchel & D. C. Turk (Eds.), *Psychological approaches to pain management: A practitioner's handbook* (pp. 131–147). New York: Guilford Press.

Bradley, L. A., Haile, J., & Jaworski, T. M. (1992). Assessment of psychological status using interviews and self-report instruments. In D. C. Turk & R. Melzack (Eds.), *Handbook of pain assessment* (pp. 235–253). New York: Guilford Press.

Butcher, J. N., Dahlstrom, W. G., Graham, J. R., Tellegen, A., & Kaemmer, B. (1989). *MMPI-2: An administrative and interpretive guide*. Minneapolis: University of Minnesota Press.

Cohen, S., & Rodriguez, M. S. (1996). Pathways linking affective disturbance and physical disorders. *Health Psychology, 14,* 374–380.

Drossman, D. A., Leserman, J., Nachman, G., Zhiming, L., Gluck, H., Toomey, T. C., & Mitchell, C. M. (1990). Sexual and physical abuse in women with functional or organic gastrointestinal disorders. *Annals of Internal Medicine, 113,* 828–833.

Dutton, M. A., Haywood, Y., & El-Bayoumi, G. (1997). Impact of violence on women's health. In S. J. Galant, G. P. Keita, & R. Royak-Schaler (Eds.), *Health care for women: Psychological, social, and behavioral influences* (pp. 41–56). Washington, DC: American Psychological Association.

Ehlert, U., Gaab, J., & Heinrichs, M. (2001). Psychoneuroendocrinological contributions to the etiology of depression, posttraumatic stress disorder, and stress-related bodily disorders: The role of the hypothalamic–pituitary–adrenal axis. *Biological Psychiatry, 57,* 141–152.

Fields, H. L. (2000). Pain modulation: Expectation, opioid analgesia, and virtual pain. *Progress in Brain Research, 122,* 245–253.

Foa, E. B., Riggs, D. S., Dancu, C. V., & Rothbaum, B. O. (1993). Reliability and validity of a brief instrument for assessing post-traumatic stress disorder. *Journal of Traumatic Stress, 6,* 459–473.

Foa, E. B., & Rothbaum, B. O. (1998). *Treating the trauma of rape: Cognitive–behavioral therapy for PTSD*. New York: Guilford Press.

Foy, D. W., Resnick, H. S., Sipprelle, R. C., & Carroll, E. M. (1987). Premilitary, military, and postmilitary factors in the development of combat related posttraumatic stress disorder. *The Behavior Therapist, 10,* 3–9.

Friedman, L. S., Samet, J. H., Roberts, M. S., & Hans, P. (1992). Inquiry about victimization experiences: A survey of patient preferences and physician practices. *Archives of Internal Medicine, 24,* 283–287.

Gatchel, R. J., & Turk, D. C. (1996). *Psychological approaches to pain management: A practitioner's handbook*. New York: Guilford Press.

Geisser, M. E., Roth, R. S., Bachman, J. E., & Eckert, T. A. (1996). The relationship between symptoms of posttraumatic stress disorder and pain, affective disturbance, and disability among patients with accident and non-accident related pain. *Pain, 66,* 207–214.

Gondolf, E. W. (1998). *Assessing woman battering in mental health services*. London: Sage.

Horowitz, M. J., Wilner, N., Alvarez, W. (1979). Impact of event scale: A measure of subjective stress. *Psychosomatic Medicine, 41,* 209–218.

Kerns, R. D., & Jacob, M. C. (1992). Assessment of the psychosocial context of the experience of chronic pain. In D. C. Turk & R. Melzack (Eds.), *Handbook of pain assessment* (pp. 235–253). New York: Guilford Press.

Lampe, A., Solder, E., Ennemoser, A., Schubert, C., Rumpold, G., & Sollner, W. (2000). Chronic pelvic pain and previous sexual abuse. *Obstetrics and Gynecology, 96,* 929–933.

Lautenbacher, S., Spernal, J., Schreiber, W., & Krieg, W. (1999). Relationship between clinical pain complaints and pain sensitivity in patients with depression and panic disorder. *Psychosomatic Medicine, 61,* 822–827.

Leserman, J., Drossman, D. A., Li, Z., Toomey, T. C., Nachman, G., & Glogau, L. (1996). Sexual and physical abuse in gastroenterology practice: How types of abuse impact health status. *Psychosomatic Medicine, 58,* 4–15.

Linton, S. J. (1997). A population-based study of the relationship between sexual abuse and back pain: Establishing a link. *Pain, 73,* 47–53.

McEwen, B. S. (2000). The neurobiology of stress: From serendipity to clinical relevance. *Brain Research, 886,* 172–189.

Meaney, M. J. (2001). Maternal care, gene expression, and the transmission of individual differences in stress reactivity across generations. *Annual Review of Neuroscience, 24,* 1161–1192.

Melzack, R., & Katz, J. (1992). The McGill Pain Questionnaire: Appraisal and current status. In D. C. Turk & R. Melzack (Eds.), *Handbook of pain assessment* (pp. 235–253). New York: Guilford Press.

Melzack, R., & Wall, P. D. (1965). Pain mechanisms: A new theory. *Science, 150,* 971–979.

Millon, T., Green, C., & Meagher, R. (1982). *Millon behavioral health inventory manual.* Minneapolis, MN: National Computer Systems.

North, R. B., Campbell, J. N., & James, C. S. (1991). Failed back surgery syndrome: 5-year follow-up in 102 patients undergoing repeated operation. *Neurosurgery, 28,* 685–690.

Resnick, H. S., Kilpatrick, D. G., Dansky, B., Saunders, B. E., & Best, C. L. (1993). Prevalence of civilian trauma in posttraumatic stress disorder in a representative national sample of women. *Journal of Consulting and Clinical Psychology, 61,* 984–991.

Rhudy, J. L., & Meagher, M. W. (2001). The role of emotion in pain modulation. *Current Opinion in Psychiatry, 14,* 241–245.

Rosen, J. B., & Schulkin, J. (1998). From normal fear to pathological anxiety. *Psychological Bulletin, 105,* 325–350.

Ruda, M. A., Ling, Q. D., Hohmann, A.G., Peng, A. G., Yuan, B., & Tachibana, T. (2000, July 28). Altered nociceptive neuronal circuits after neonatal peripheral inflammation. *Science, 289,* 628–630.

Scarinci, I. C., McDonald-Haile, J., Bradley, L. A., & Richter, J. E. (1994). Altered pain perception and psychosocial features among women with gastrointestinal disorders and history of abuse: A preliminary model. *American Journal of Medicine, 97,* 108–118.

Schofferman, J., Anderson, D., Hinds, R., Smith, G., & White, A. (1992). Childhood psychological trauma correlates with unsuccessful lumbar spine surgery. *Spine, 17*, S1381–S1384.

Sharp, T. J., & Harvey, A. G. (2001). Chronic pain and posttraumatic stress disorder: Mutual maintenance? *Clinical Psychology Review, 21*, 857–877.

Shors, T. J., Weiss, C., & Thompson, R. F. (1992, July 24). Stress-induced facilitation of classical conditioning. *Science, 257*, 537–539.

Spertus, I. L., Burns, J., Glenn, B., Lofland, K., & McCracken, L. (1999). Gender differences in associations between trauma history and adjustment among chronic pain patients. *Pain, 82*, 97–102.

Stephan, M., Helfritz, F., Pabst, R., & von Horsten, S. (2002). Postnatally induced differences in adult pain sensitivity depend on genetics, gender, and specific experiences: Reversal of maternal deprivation effects by additional postnatal tactile stimulation or chronic imipramine treatment. *Behavioral Brain Research, 133*, 149–158.

True, W. R., Rice, J., Eisen, S. A., Heath, A. C., Goldberg, J., Lyons, M. J., & Nowak, J. (1993). A twin study of genetic and environmental contributions to liability for posttraumatic stress symptoms. *Archives of General Psychiatry, 50*, 257–264.

Turk, D. C. (1995, August). *Chronic pain > physical disease: Psychological contributions to rehabilitation and cost savings.* Paper presented at the Presidential Miniconvention, "To Your Health: Psychology Through the Life Span," at the 103rd Annual Convention of the American Psychological Association, New York.

Turk, D. C. (1996). Biopsychosocial perspectives on chronic pain. In R. J. Gatchel & D. C. Turk (Eds.), *Psychological approaches to pain management: A practitioner's handbook* (pp. 3–32). New York: Guilford Press.

Turk, D. C., Meichenbaum, D., & Genest, M. (1983). *Pain and behavioral medicine: A cognitive–behavioral perspective.* New York: Guilford Press.

Turk, D. C., & Melzack, R. (1992). *Handbook of pain assessment.* New York: Guilford Press.

van der Kolk, B. A., Pelcovitz, D., Roth, S., Mandel, F. S., McFarlane, A., & Herman J. L. (1996). Dissociation, somatization, and affect dysregulation: The complexity of adaptation to trauma. *American Journal of Psychiatry, 153*, 83–93.

Vernberg, E. M., La Greca, A. M., Silverman, W. K., & Prinstein, M. J. (1996). Prediction of posttraumatic stress symptoms in children after Hurricane Andrew. *Journal of Abnormal Psychology, 105*, 235–248.

Waddell, G. (1987). Volvo award in clinical sciences: A new clinical model for the treatment of low-back pain. *Spine, 12*, 632–644.

Walker, E. A., Gelfand, A., Katon, W. J., Koss, M. P., Von Korff, M., Bernstein, D., & Russo, J. (1999). Adult health status of women with histories of childhood abuse and neglect. *American Journal of Medicine, 107*, 332–339.

Walker, E. A., Katon, W. J., Roy-Byrne, P., Jemelka, R., & Russo, J. (1993). Histories of sexual victimization in patients with irritable bowel syndrome or inflammatory bowel disease. *American Journal of Psychiatry, 150*, 1502–1506.

Walling, M. K., Reiter, R. C., O'Hara, M. W., Milburn, A. K., Lilly, G., & Vincent, S.D. (1994). Abuse history and chronic pain in women: I. Prevalences of sexual abuse and physical abuse. *Obstetrics and Gynecology, 84,* 193–199.

Watkins, L. R., & Maier, S. F. (2000). The pain of being sick: Implications of immune-to-brain communication for understanding pain. *Annual Review of Psychology, 51,* 29–57.

Woolf, C. J., & Mannion, R. J. (1999). Neuropathic pain: Aetiology, symptoms, mechanisms, and management. *The Lancet, 353,* 1959–1964.

10

VICTIMIZATION AND HEALTH RISK BEHAVIORS: IMPLICATIONS FOR PREVENTION PROGRAMS

JOANNE L. DAVIS, AMY M. COMBS-LANE, AND DANIEL W. SMITH

Even the best prevention programs have clients they cannot reach. Clinicians conducting prevention programs often find that the people who persist in risky behavior have had abuse experiences. Results from research studies have been striking. Research indicates that victims of trauma in general, and family violence in particular, report greater involvement in a number of health risk behaviors than nonvictims. This finding is consistent across different types of family violence (e.g., sexual abuse, physical abuse) and is particularly salient for victims who have experienced multiple incidents. Health risk behaviors that have been examined empirically include alcohol consumption, lack of exercise or inactivity, illicit drug use, tobacco use, eating disorders, sexual activity with numerous partners, sexual intercourse early in a relationship, failure to use contraceptives, and sexual activity while under the influence of alcohol or drugs. Research further suggests that unless these traumatic events are addressed, prevention and treatment efforts are likely to fail.

Health risk behaviors are responsible for the most serious social and health problems in the United States (Centers for Disease Control and Prevention, n.d.). Because of higher rates of involvement in health risk behaviors, victims of family violence are at a significantly greater risk than nonvictims for a variety of acute and chronic health problems, including violence-related injury, suicide, HIV infection or other sexually transmitted diseases, unintended pregnancy, development of chronic disease related to substance use, and revictimization. Despite the increased recognition of this phenomenon, knowledge is lacking with respect to why victims of family violence report greater involvement in health risk behaviors. This is an obstacle for mental and physical health providers who attempt to prevent or reduce victims' involvement in these behaviors.

Before we describe the current status and implications of health risk behaviors and family violence, a few caveats are necessary. First, in terms of child abuse experiences, the majority of research has been conducted with survivors of child sexual abuse; far less has looked at survivors of physical abuse, neglect, or individuals who have witnessed family violence. However, these other forms of maltreatment often co-occur with sexual abuse and are therefore studied indirectly. Furthermore, whereas child sexual abuse, physical abuse, neglect, and the witnessing of familial violence are typically assumed to be perpetrated by a parental figure, sexual assault is more frequently perpetrated by someone outside the family. Nonfamilial sexual assault can lead to many of the same health risk behaviors. Research conducted on the involvement in and the prevention and treatment of health risk behaviors typically has not distinguished between victims of familial and nonfamilial violence. These limitations are similar to the broader field of research on the negative correlates of family violence and trauma (e.g., depression, anxiety disorders; e.g., see Jumper, 1995). Thus, although these limitations are not unique to research on health risk behaviors, they do reflect gaps in current knowledge of family violence. Future research will need to address these concerns. However, the body of research is large enough for us to make suggestions for working with survivors now.

In this chapter we provide an overview of health risk behaviors and related acute and chronic diseases associated with a history of family violence. We begin with a brief review of the research on the involvement of family violence victims in health risk behaviors. Next, we provide a brief description of the acute and chronic physical health problems related to health risk behaviors. Then we describe assessment of health risk behaviors and related mental health concerns, followed by information on treatment and prevention interventions. At the end of the chapter, we provide a list of resources (see Appendix A) for further information.

SCREENING FOR HEALTH RISK BEHAVIORS

Asking abuse survivors questions about health risk behaviors (e.g., "Were you drinking at the time of the assault?" "Do you drink often?") may be perceived as victim-blaming and thus may be uncomfortable for clinicians.

Because of feelings of shame or guilt, victims may not be forthcoming about either their traumatic experiences or their involvement in health risk behaviors. However, given the risks to physical and mental health and the clients' safety, it is important that both mental and physical health care providers address these issues.

To initiate a discussion of health risk behaviors, clinicians may want to ask about coping strategies and tension reduction behaviors ("Is there anything that you do that helps you to feel better or forget about the trauma?"). For several areas of health risk behaviors, a structured clinical interview (e.g., the Structured Clinical Interview for the *Diagnostic and Statistical Manual of Mental Disorders* [DSM–IV]; American Psychiatric Association, 1994; First, Spitzer, Gibbon, & Williams, 1996) will provide information on criteria for particular disorders (e.g., substance abuse and dependence, eating disorders). Self-report instruments are also available. For instance, tension reduction behaviors and risky sexual behaviors are included on the Trauma Symptom Inventory (Briere, 1995). If urine drug screen tests are available, clinicians may use them to assess for substance use. Clinicians may also want to assess problems related to the risky behavior, including possible educational, social, interpersonal, and vocational problems. Finally, clinicians may want to assess social cognitions related to health risk behaviors. The Cognitive Appraisal of Risky Events (Fromme, Katz, & Rivet, 1997) assesses perceptions of risk and benefit associated with risky behaviors (e.g., alcohol and drug use, risky sexual activities), previous involvement in these behaviors, and behavioral intentions to engage in these same behaviors in the future.

Acute Health Care Needs

For victims of recent family violence, a number of health-related factors must first be addressed before clinicians can target health risk behaviors. The adverse effects of many health risk behaviors unfortunately are often not fully evident until much later. Thus, certain health-related factors are often overlooked until they develop into significant problems. In the early stages of treatment, mental health providers can be helpful in providing accurate information, making recommendations for medical follow-up, and assisting victims in obtaining appropriate medical care monitoring to ensure that victims follow through with treatment recommendations. Support and encouragement are particularly important, because the majority of assault victims do not receive standard medical care after an assault (R. F. Hanson et al., 2001; Resnick, Holmes, et al., 2000) or do not return for follow-up visits in which important education and prevention information is often provided (Holmes, Resnick, & Frampton, 1998). This is particularly important for child victims of family violence, as they are unable to obtain this care themselves and parents may not seek medical care for them. For example, R. F. Hanson et al. (2001) found that 96% of victims of intrafamilial rape did not receive a medical examination after the assault.

After sexual and physical assaults, injuries to the face, head, neck, legs, inner thighs, genitals, breasts, upper extremities, and torso are common (Koss & Heslet, 1992; Resnick, Acierno, & Kilpatrick, 1997; Sommers, Schafer, Zink, Hutson, & Hillard, 2001). Less frequently, victims experience fractures, internal injuries, and head injuries that require more extensive medical interventions (Kilpatrick, Edmunds, & Seymour, 1992). It is also important to discuss issues related to sexually transmitted diseases (STDs), HIV, and pregnancy early in treatment, particularly for individuals who have experienced sexual assault. Data indicate that rape victims have higher rates of STDs compared with nonvictims (Irwin et al., 1995) and are frequently concerned about the possibility of having contracted HIV due to rape (R. F. Hanson et al., 2001; Kilpatrick et al., 1992; Resnick, Acierno, Holmes, Dammeyer, & Kilpatrick, 2000). Holmes, Resnick, Kilpatrick, and Best (1996) reported that 5% of rape victims in the National Women's Study had experienced an unintended pregnancy as a result of their rape.

In addition to ensuring that individuals obtain appropriate medical care, it is important to address psychological aspects of functioning that may contribute to physical health problems and engagement in health risk behaviors. Victims of family violence report increased psychological distress and mental health problems that may have profound effects on physical health. For example, a growing literature suggests that symptoms of posttraumatic stress disorder (PTSD) may play a motivating role in the onset and maintenance of health risk behaviors. Indeed, Kilpatrick and colleagues (1992) noted that "PTSD is clearly an independent risk factor for virtually all of the negative mental and physical health consequences of violence" (p. 80). Other diagnoses and conditions associated with experiencing family violence include additional anxiety disorders (e.g., panic disorder), mood disorders (e.g., depression), and interpersonal problems (e.g., difficulty trusting others). In addition, research has identified systemic changes associated with a history of trauma and high levels of chronic stress, including impaired immune system functioning (Resnick et al., 1997) and alterations in brain functioning (Yehuda, Giller, Southwick, Lowry, & Mason, 1991). Psychosocial interventions designed to lower psychological distress have been found to provide health benefits (Pennebaker, 1999).

Long-Term Health Care Needs

Health risk behaviors may place family violence victims at increased risk for chronic health problems. The association between health risk behaviors and chronic illness in victims of family violence may be due to a number of factors. First, victims may have engaged in the health risk behavior for a long period of time before receiving treatment from a mental or physical health care provider. Compared with other types of violence, violence occurring in the family is typically characterized by earlier onset, greater frequency, and longer duration. Thus, the coping strategies embraced by victims may start at a relatively young age and continue through the course of the abuse. Moreover, the chronic nature of family violence may heighten the level of distress, increasing the use of maladaptive coping strategies. By the time the violence has ended, the behaviors may be deeply engrained in the developmental mindset of the victim. The behaviors often continue well past the end of the abuse (indeed, they may not begin until after the abuse has ended), in part because of the negative reinforcing qualities of the behaviors.

Second, the potential adverse health effects of the behaviors may be easily dismissed, particularly by adolescents, as they are often not evident until later in life. Third, involvement in health risk behaviors may contribute to other problems in life, including poor performance in school and work, interpersonal difficulties, and legal problems. This may result in increased stress and mental health problems that could potentially impair the client's immune functioning and further increase the risk of physical health problems. Fourth, health risk behaviors are often used as a means of escaping or avoiding negative cognitions, affect, and memories related to the trauma. Health risk behaviors may also help a person avoid dealing with acute trauma-related physical problems, resulting in long-term physical problems (Resnick et al., 1997).

Regardless of an individual's trauma history, health risk behaviors are associated with high rates of relapse and recidivism. Because victims of family violence face a number of additional psychosocial and health-related challenges, it may be particularly difficult for them to maintain positive changes. Numerous attempts may be required for permanent behavioral changes. Factors such as an individual's learning history, current psychological distress, ongoing abuse, coping abilities, access to resources, and motivation may affect an individual's ability to resist engaging in health risk behaviors and need to be considered in planning treatment and prevention efforts.

It is unfortunate that certain types of health risk behaviors may result in chronic and potentially fatal conditions (e.g., AIDS, ischemic heart disease, cancer, lung disease, skeletal fractures, liver damage) even after the behavior has stopped. The nature and course of any illness of course depends on numerous factors, including gender, ethnicity, genetic propensity, and other lifestyle factors. Moreover, women may experience additional health problems, including fertility problems, pregnancy complications, and increased rates of cervical cancer. Chances of recovery from these conditions vary on the basis of the nature of the condition, duration, and extent of involvement in the health risk behavior; other physical and mental health difficulties; access to and appropriate use of medical services; and other life stressors.

STRATEGIES FOR ADDRESSING HEALTH RISK BEHAVIORS

General Strategies

The strategies outlined below are intended as general guidelines for intervening with victims engaging in health risk behaviors. A number of treatment packages are available that focus on specific health risk behaviors; many of these have empirical support. Some of these treatment manuals are included in the resources section at the end of this chapter.

Psychoeducation

Psychoeducation should be a part of any intervention targeting health risk behaviors. Mental health providers can begin by providing information about behaviors that are associated with risk for health-related problems and future victimization. Although clinicians should be cautious to avoid statements that may be perceived as victim-blaming in nature, they can assist individuals in evaluating the pros and cons of various behaviors and discussing the victim's behavioral intentions to engage in particular health risk behaviors (Combs-Lane & Smith, 2002).

Clinicians may also address emotion regulation processes with individuals who are avoidant of negative affect (Cloitre, 1998; Polusny & Follette, 1995). This may involve identifying and labeling emotions, determining ways to appropriately express emotions, and conducting exposure therapy to trauma cues associated with the negative emotions. Clients can be provided instruction on alternative coping strategies to assist them in dealing with negative affect and memories of the trauma. Strategies such as progressive muscle relaxation, breathing retraining, guided imagery, building a support network, and improving self-care may decrease an individual's motivation for involvement with health risk behaviors

It may also be beneficial to assess the victim's perceptions of health risk behaviors. Research indicates that identifying, challenging, and modifying distorted cognitions may be particularly important in altering health risk behaviors. Victims and nonvictims often differ in their assessments of the risks and benefits involved in health risk behaviors. Smith and colleagues (2002) assessed judgments of risks and benefits of four categories of health risk behaviors: (a) illicit drug use, (b) risky sexual behaviors, (c) aggressive or illegal behaviors, and (d) heavy drinking. They found that victims rated illicit drug use and risky sexual behaviors as less risky and more beneficial than did nonvictims. There are many possible explanations for the results that have implications for treatment. First, victims may lack education regarding the risks and benefits of health risk behaviors. Second, victims may be aware of the potential for negative consequences and have even experienced some negative consequences of their behaviors. However, they may be focusing on the short-term benefits of escape/avoidance of trauma-related memories and emotions. Third, victims' ratings may reflect their experiences with the behavior. Research indicates that risk ratings decrease as experience with the behavior increases (e.g., DiLillo, Potts, & Himes, 1998). The clinician will need to determine the client's perceptions of the behaviors to intervene appropriately.

Behavioral Strategies

Often behavioral strategies are used to alter levels of engagement in health risk behaviors. Treatment may involve identifying maladaptive behaviors, determining the factors that maintain the behaviors, identifying alternative behaviors that are more adaptive, and increasing involvement in the alternative behaviors. Power, esteem, safety, trust, and intimacy are areas commonly affected by trauma (McCann, Sakheim, & Abrahamson, 1988), and difficulties in these areas may be part of the victim's underlying motivation for engaging in health risk behaviors. For example, a woman may engage in risky sexual behaviors to feel a sense of power and control over men. Interventions that focus on the removal of these maladaptive behaviors are unlikely to be successful if the underlying motivation is not considered. It is important to identify the perceived benefits of the risk behaviors so that treatment can focus on replacing the behavior while maintaining the benefits. In addition to decreasing health risk behaviors, clinicians can also assist clients in increasing health care behaviors. Education and behavioral strategies can focus on increasing obtaining regular Pap smears, regular physical checkups, increasing one's physical activity level, and proper nutrition.

Addressing Self-Blame

Health risk behaviors can increase the risk of revictimization. Victims may be concerned that the clinician will judge them harshly or negatively if they disclose past or current involvement in health risk behaviors. If the victim engaged in health risk behaviors prior to or during the incident, feelings of guilt and shame may be present. Clinicians need to assess for feelings of self-blame directly. It may be appropriate to ask victims why they believe the assault occurred, whom they feel was responsible, and if they believe there was anything that could have prevented it from occurring. Clinicians need to be aware that victims often feel a sense of personal responsibility and, at the same time, be aware that self-blame is associated with poorer outcomes. Thus, one consequence of self-blame is that it may interfere with an individual's ability to address health risk behaviors. In this event, it is necessary to first address the cognitive processes associated with guilt and self-blame.

Adjunct Services

With respect to targeting health risk behaviors in treatment, health care providers, including mental health providers, may want to refer clients for adjunct services. For instance, a physical or gynecological examination, substance abuse evaluation and treatment, or testing for STDs and HIV may be appropriate. Before making a referral, clinicians are advised to address factors related to the client's comfort and willingness to comply with the recommendation. Clients may have specific requests of the referral source that will enable them to feel more comfortable (e.g., meeting with the provider ahead of time). The clinician can assist the client in making specific arrangements to ensure the visit proceeds according to plans. In some cases, it may be helpful to have someone accompany the individual to the appointment. Rape crisis centers and domestic violence shelters often have trained advocates who can accompany victims during health care visits.

Mental health providers are ideally in the best position to help victims of family violence when they can establish a network of connections with professionals in the community. It is useful to identify all types of providers who have experience working with victims of family violence and are committed to providing a safe environment in which victim issues are appropriately addressed. An ideal network includes specially trained physicians and nurses who perform physical and gynecological evaluations, law enforcement agencies that provide advocacy services to victims of crime, community agencies that offer a broad array of victim services, and mental health providers who have specialized training in the area of trauma and violence.

Trauma-Focused Interventions

In addition to the above strategies, clinicians need to specifically address the trauma caused by past or current abuse. A number of treatment strategies have been shown to be effective in alleviating the mental health consequences of the trauma, in particular, PTSD. Manualized treatments with published support for their efficacy include cognitive processing therapy (Resick & Schnicke, 1993), prolonged exposure (Foa & Rothbaum, 1998), stress inoculation training (Kilpatrick, Veronen, & Resick, 1982), and multiple channel exposure therapy (Falsetti, Resnick, & Davis, in press; Falsetti & Resnick, 2000). The impact of these treatments on health risk behaviors is unknown, however, because many treatment outcome studies exclude individuals who engage in high-risk behaviors, including substance use, or do not include health risk behaviors as outcome variables. Furthermore, as noted above, current research does not distinguish between victims of family violence and victims of other violence. However, these issues can be addressed in future research.

Prioritizing Treatment Goals

It is rare to encounter any client with just one difficulty or issue; victims of family violence often report numerous mental and physical health problems. Clinicians may feel somewhat overwhelmed by the number of issues and magnitude of distress reported by these individuals. Prioritizing targets of treatment in these cases is challenging. Clinicians may question whether it is necessary to first target specific psychological symptoms, in an attempt to decrease the related negative affect, avoidance behaviors, and maladaptive cognitions associated with the trauma, or whether it is appropriate to focus first on the health risk behaviors in an effort to reduce negative health consequences and the client's risk for revictimization. Clinicians should ask themselves some questions, such as the following: Which approach is likely to be better tolerated by the client? Furthermore, with respect to interventions for health risk behaviors, what are the best treatment approaches with victims of family violence? Do these differ from standard approaches with victims of nonfamily violence or nonvictims? To attempt to answer these questions, we turn to the literature pertaining to victimization and substance abuse because substance-related health risk behaviors are the most frequently discussed in the victimization literature.

Research findings indicate a significant association between substance abuse and PTSD (Dansky, Saladin, Brady, Kilpatrick, & Resnick, 1995; Najavits, Weiss, & Shaw, 1997). Also, both are common sequelae of childhood abuse. The combination of the two disorders is marked by a higher level of social impairment, poorer treatment outcome, more severe symptoms, and higher rates of other pathology than either disorder alone (Brady, Dansky, Back, Foa, & Carroll, 2001; Najavits, Weiss, Shaw, & Muenz, 1998). Traditional forms of treatment for either disorder alone may be ineffective and even contraindicated for individuals suffering from both problems. For example, PTSD symptoms have been found to increase with abstinence, whereas other comorbid Axis I disorders tend to remit with abstinence (Najavits et al., 1997).

Several different approaches to addressing the issue of the comorbidity of PTSD and substance abuse have been discussed. Arguments have been made for treating the disorders separately and consecutively, whereas other researchers advocate for concurrent and simultaneous treatment. In a comprehensive review of the treatment of PTSD and substance use, Ruzek, Polusny, and Abueg (1998) argued against the simultaneous treatment of PTSD and substance abuse and stated that substance abuse issues need to be addressed before PTSD symptoms are treated. They theorized that individuals seeking treatment, when not treated for their substance abuse issues first, are limited in their ability to use healthy coping strategies, gain support from their social network, and engage in trauma-focused treatment; they also have an increased vulnerability to experiencing other trauma or victimization because of their substance-induced impairment. Zaslav (1994) discussed ways in which substance abuse may interfere with PTSD treatment, including how substance abusers may have difficulty sustaining a commitment to psychotherapy and maintaining the therapeutic alliance. In addition, individuals with substance abuse problems may have difficulty tolerating negative affect associated with addressing the trauma, which may result in relapse or dropout from treatment (Beck, Wright, Newman, & Liese, 1993).

Alternatively, others have argued for the simultaneous treatment of substance abuse and PTSD (e.g., Kofoed, Friedman, & Peck, 1993). This perspective suggests that if trauma issues and PTSD symptoms are not addressed early on in treatment, negative affect will continue, lessening the likelihood that substance use will decrease and increasing the chance of dropout and relapse. Also, if the motivation for substance use is in part to reduce negative affect and trauma-related memories, then addressing the PTSD symptoms early on may decrease the client's perceived need for substance use. The simultaneous treatment of PTSD and substance abuse has recently received more attention; several manualized treatments have been published, including "Concurrent Treatment of PTSD and Cocaine Dependence" (Back, Dansky, Carroll, Foa, & Brady, 2001), "Seeking Safety" (Najavits et al., 1998), and "Substance Dependence PTSD Therapy" (Triffleman, Carroll, & Kellogg, 1999). Although more research is necessary to draw firm conclusions, it appears that typical treatments of either disorder are unlikely to be effective in meeting the needs of this population. This is likely to be true for victims of family violence who engage in other types of health risk behaviors as well.

What does this mean for clinicians who work primarily or extensively with victims of family violence? First, clinicians need to recognize and understand the implications of working with clients who engage in health risk behaviors. Second, the nature and course of treatment need to be adapted to meet the unique needs of victims who are struggling with both health risk behaviors and other consequences of family violence. Third, it is important for clinicians to understand that both trauma symptoms and health risk behaviors are well established patterns for the client, and thus treatment may take several attempts. Fourth, clinicians working with victims of family violence who are not familiar with treatment of addictions and other health risk behaviors may want to seek additional training and supervision, particularly focusing on evidence-based treatments for these comorbid conditions. Alternatively, it is possible that treatment may be effective if conducted separately, but concurrently (see Davis, Davies, Wright, Roitzsch, & Falsetti, in press). In this case, the clinician may want to establish a good working relationship with a colleague who specializes in treating the health risk behavior in question and work together with him or her to meet the needs of the client.

Although this discussion has focused on substance use, the treatment issues described may be relevant for other types of risk-taking behaviors. In fact, the substance use–PTSD treatments described above also include modules targeting other risk-taking behaviors (Back et al., 2001; Triffleman et al., 1999). For example, "Concurrent Treatment of PTSD and Cocaine Dependence" (Back et al., 2001) includes an HIV module. Back et al. list the following as primary goals of this module: (a) educate about HIV testing, transmission, and prevention; (b) increase sexual assertiveness behaviors; and (c) decrease HIV high-risk behaviors. Outcome data specific to HIV-related behaviors unfortunately were not provided in the studies.

PREVENTION EFFORTS

Secondary prevention programs are those that target individuals who have been victimized; the aim of such programs is to reduce the negative consequences of the victimization. Numerous investigations have examined interventions designed to change health risk behaviors, reduce the negative impact of health risk behaviors, or prevent involvement in these behaviors. Research indicates that although many interventions are effective in meeting these goals, few of these investigations report results by victimization status. As we mentioned earlier, the results of evaluations of programs or treatments indicate that victims may not be as amenable to reducing health risk behaviors as nonvictims. Because of space limitations, we cannot address treatments available for all health risk behaviors; instead, we briefly review those that were developed specifically for victims of trauma. First, we review two treatments that target substance dependence and PTSD. Second, we review two broad-based prevention programs aimed at reducing the risk of dating violence (for victims and nonvictims of previous violence), in part, through a focus on health risk behaviors. None of these studies, however, distinguishes victims of family violence and other types of violence.

Treatment Outcome Studies

Although there are currently three manualized treatments targeting comorbid substance use and PTSD, only two have published results of the treatment outcome studies (Brady et al., 2001; Najavits et al., 1998). Najavits et al. (1998) examined the efficacy of a group cognitive–behavioral treatment developed to treat both PTSD and substance dependence, called "Seeking Safety." Seeking Safety focuses on cognitive, behavioral, and interpersonal domains. Seventeen (of 27) women completed the treatment. Results indicated that treatment completers reported decreased substance use that was maintained through the follow-up assessment at three months. Although PTSD symptoms were not significantly reduced at posttreatment, they were significantly lower at the follow-up assessment. Najavits et al. reported that this finding was not surprising, as PTSD symptoms may not ameliorate during the initial phase of abstinence. This study unfortunately did not include a control group, so the treatment's comparative efficacy is unknown. Moreover, the follow-up period was relatively short. In spite of these limitations, the study showed promise for a new treatment specifically tailored for women with both PTSD and substance dependence.

Brady et al. (2001) evaluated 15 men and women who met criteria for both PTSD and cocaine dependence. The dropout rate for this study was 62%. Significant differences between completers and noncompleters included lower education and higher avoidance for noncompleters. Analysis of the completers indicated that the treatment was effective in reducing symptoms of PTSD and substance use severity. These gains were maintained through the follow-up period at six months. It is interesting that Brady et al. also reported that exposure treatment did not appear to precipitate dropout or relapse to drug use. Limitations of this study include the small sample size, lack of a control group, and a high dropout rate.

There appears to be some efficacy for the use of these treatments that were specially developed or modified treatments for victims of violence. The process by which these treatments were modified from standard treatments for both PTSD and substance use may serve as models for treatments already in use with other health risk behaviors (e.g., eating disorders, smoking). Much research is needed to determine the efficacy of other evidence-based treatments with victims of violence and victims of family violence in particular.

Prevention Program Outcome Studies

The literature on broad-based prevention programs designed to reduce involvement in health risk behaviors mirrors that described above for disorder-specific treatments. A number of programs have shown efficacy in reducing involvement in health risk behaviors (see the Web site of the Centers for Disease Control and Prevention for an overview of many of these programs: http://www.cdc.gov/nccdphp/dash/rtc/index.htm). The majority of these programs are school- or community-based interventions targeting middle and high school students. These programs appear to be effective in improving knowledge of various health risk behaviors, reducing risky sexual activities (e.g., having intercourse with fewer partners), increasing safe sexual behaviors (e.g., wearing a condom during intercourse), reducing unintentional pregnancy, and decreasing smoking behavior. Again, these programs may be potentially applicable to victims of family violence. However, few investigations have evaluated efficacy by victimization status. We are aware of two prevention programs that specifically addressed health risk behaviors and evaluated the outcome by victimization status (although neither distinguished between family and nonfamily violence; Davis, Jackson, & DeMaio, 1998; Hanson-Breitenbecher & Gidycz, 1998).

Hanson-Breitenbecher and Gidycz (1998) implemented a sexual assault prevention program with college women that focused on potentially risky dating behaviors and sexual communication (K. A. Hanson & Gidycz, 1993). These investigators found that although awareness of sexual assault increased after the program, the incidence of victimization was not reduced, and no changes were reported in dating behaviors and sexual communication for both victims and nonvictims of previous assaults. Davis et al. (1998) conducted a similar study that included a sexual assault education and prevention program for college women, with a specific target on health risk behaviors, including risky sexual behaviors (e.g., sleeping with someone one has just met), substance use (e.g., drinking to the point of passing out), and general risk behaviors (e.g., walking alone late at night). Results indicated that knowledge of sexual assault issues was increased at the three-month follow-up. However, involvement in health risk behaviors did not change for victims or nonvictims of violence.

CONCLUSION

Although some prevention programs have had positive results, many have not. The finding that broad-based prevention programs have generally failed to establish lasting changes in behavior is not restricted to those that target victims of family violence. In a discourse on the efficacy of peer health education at colleges and universities, Fabiano (1994) stated that "evidence exists that critical health behavior change in students' real, everyday lives has not followed from gains in their knowledge, shifts in their attitudes and beliefs, or acquisition of new skills" (p. 115). Although the problem of changing health risk behaviors extends beyond victims of family violence, different approaches may be needed when trying to change the behaviors of this specific population. Prevention programmers need to consider alternate approaches that bear in mind the particular issues faced by victims of family violence.

ADDITIONAL RESOURCES

Centers for Disease Control and Prevention, *Programs That Work*. Available: http://www.cdc.gov/nccdphp/dash/rtc/index.htm

Duberstein Lindberg, L., Boggess, S., Porter, L., & Williams, S. (2000). Teen risk-taking: A statistical portrait. Available: http://www.urban.org/family/teenrisktaking.html

Gottheil, E. L. (1999). *Effects of substance abuse treatment on AIDS risk behaviors.* Binghamton, NY: Haworth.

Heise, L., Ellsberg, M., & Gottemoeller, M. (1999, December). *Ending violence against women: Population reports* (Population Information Program, Series L, No. 11). Baltimore: Johns Hopkins University School of Public Health. Available: http://www.jhuccp.org/pr/l11/l11chap5_1.stm

Lerner, R. M. (1995). *America's youth in crisis: Challenges and options for programs and policies.* Thousand Oaks, CA: Sage.

Lightfoot, C. (1997). *The culture of adolescent risk taking.* New York: Guilford Press.

Lipsitt, L. P., & Mitnick, L. L. (Eds.). (1991). *Self regulatory behavior and risk taking: Causes and consequences.* Portland, OR: Book News.

National Institute on Drug Abuse, (n.d.). Advances in Research on Women's Health and Gender Differences. Available: http://165.112.78.61/whgd/whgdadvance.html

REFERENCES

American Psychiatric Association. (1994). *Diagnostic and statistical manual of mental disorders* (4th ed.). Washington, DC: Author.

Back, S. E., Dansky, B. S., Carroll, K. M., Foa, E. B., & Brady, K. T. (2001). Exposure therapy in the treatment of PTSD among cocaine-dependent individuals: Description of the procedures. *Journal of Substance Abuse Treatment, 21*, 35–45.

Beck, A. T., Wright, F. D., Newman, C. F., & Liese, B. S. (1993). *Cognitive therapy of substance abuse.* New York: Guilford Press.

Brady, K. T., Dansky, B. S., Back, S. E., Foa, E. B., & Carroll, K. M. (2001). Exposure therapy in the treatment of PTSD among cocaine-dependent individuals: Preliminary findings. *Journal of Substance Abuse Treatment, 21*, 47–54.

Briere, J. (1995). *Professional manual for the Trauma Symptom Inventory.* Odessa, FL: Psychological Assessment Resources.

Centers for Disease Control and Prevention. (n.d.). *Adolescent and school health.* Retrieved February 2, 2002, from http://www.cdc.gov/nccdphp/dash/risk.htm

Cloitre, M. (1998). Sexual revictimization: Risk factors and prevention. In V. M. Follette, J. I. Ruzek, & F. R. Abueg (Eds.), *Cognitive–behavioral therapies for trauma* (pp. 278–304). New York: Guilford Press.

Combs-Lane, A. M., & Smith, D. W. (2002). Risk of sexual victimization in college women: The role of behavioral intentions and risk-taking behaviors. *Journal of Interpersonal Violence, 17,* 165–183.

Dansky, B. S., Saladin, M. E., Brady, K. T., Kilpatrick, D. G., & Resnick, H. S. (1995). Prevalence of victimization and posttraumatic stress disorder among women with substance use disorders: Comparison of telephone and in-person assessment samples. *International Journal of the Addictions, 30,* 1079–1099.

Davis, J. L., Davies, S., Wright, D., Roitzsch, J., & Falsetti, S. A. (in press). Simultaneous treatment of substance abuse and posttraumatic stress disorder: A case example. *Clinical Case Studies.*

Davis, J. L., Jackson, T. L., & DeMaio, C. M. (1998, November). *An empirical investigation of a sexual assault education and prevention program on knowledge, attitudes, and expected involvement in risky sexual behaviors.* Poster presented at the 32nd annual conference of the Association for Advancement of Behavior Therapy, Washington, DC.

DiLillo, D., Potts, R., & Himes, S. (1998). Predictors of children's risk appraisals. *Journal of Applied Developmental Psychology, 19,* 415–427.

Fabiano, P. M. (1994). From personal health into community action: Another step forward in peer health education. *Journal of College Health, 43,* 115–121.

Falsetti, S. A., & Resnick, H. S. (2000). Cognitive behavioral treatment for PTSD with comorbid panic attacks. *Journal of Contemporary Psychotherapy, 30,* 163–179.

Falsetti, S. A., Resnick, H. S., & Davis, J. L. (in press). Multiple channel exposure therapy: Combining cognitive behavioral therapies for the treatment of posttraumatic stress disorder with panic attacks. *Behavior Modification.*

First, M. B., Spitzer, R. L., Gibbon, M., & Williams, J. B. W. (1996). *Structured clinical interview for DSM–IV disorders.* New York: Biometrics Research Department.

Foa, E. B., & Rothbaum, B. (1998). *Treating the trauma of rape: Cognitive behavioral therapy for PTSD.* New York: Guilford Press.

Fromme, K., Katz, E. C., & Rivet, K. (1997). Outcome expectancies and risk-taking behavior. *Cognitive Therapy and Research, 21,* 421–442.

Hanson, K. A., & Gidycz, C. A. (1993). An evaluation of a sexual assault prevention program. *Journal of Consulting and Clinical Psychology, 61,* 1046–1052.

Hanson-Breitenbecher, K. A., & Gidycz, C. A. (1998). An empirical evaluation of a program designed to reduce the risk of multiple sexual victimization. *Journal of Interpersonal Violence, 13,* 472–488.

Hanson, R. F., Davis, J. L., Resnick, H. S., Saunders, B. E., Kilpatrick, D. G., Holmes, M., & Best, C. L. (2001). Predictors of medical exams following child and adolescent rapes in a national sample of women. *Child Maltreatment, 6*, 250–259.

Holmes, M. M., Resnick, H. S., & Frampton, D. (1998). Follow-up of sexual assault victims. *American Journal of Obstetrics and Gynecology, 179*, 336–342.

Holmes, M. M., Resnick, H. S., Kilpatrick, D. G., & Best, C. L. (1996). Rape-related pregnancy: Estimates and descriptive characteristics from a national sample of women. *American Journal of Obstetrics and Gynecology, 175*, 320–325.

Irwin, K. L., Edlin, B. R., Wong, L., Faruque, S., McCoy, H. V., Word, C., et al. (1995). Urban rape survivors: Characteristics and prevalence of human immunodeficiency virus and other sexually transmitted infections. *Obstetrics and Gynecology, 85*, 330–336.

Jumper, S. A. (1995). A meta-analysis of the relationship of child sexual abuse to adult psychological adjustment. *Child Abuse & Neglect, 19*, 715–728.

Kilpatrick, D. G., Edmunds, C., & Seymour, A. E. (1992). *Rape in America: A report to the nation.* Arlington, VA and Charleston, SC: National Victim Center and Crime Victims Research and Treatment Center.

Kilpatrick, D. G., Veronen, L. J., & Resick, P. A. (1982). Psychological sequelae to rape: Assessment and treatment strategies. In D. M. Dolays & R. L. Meredith (Eds.), *Behavioral medicine: Assessment and treatment strategies* (pp. 473–497). New York: Plenum.

Kofoed, M. D., Friedman, M. J., & Peck, R. (1993). Alcoholism and drug abuse in patients with PTSD. *Psychiatric Quarterly, 64*, 151–171.

Koss, M. P., & Heslet, L. (1992). Somatic consequences of violence against women. *Archives of Family Medicine, 1*, 53–59.

McCann, I. L., Sakheim, D. K., & Abrahamson, D. J. (1988). Trauma and victimization: A model of psychological adaptation. *The Counseling Psychologist, 16*, 531–594.

Najavits, L. M., Weiss, R. D., & Shaw, S. R. (1997). The link between substance abuse and posttraumatic stress disorder in women: A research review. *American Journal of Addictions, 6*, 273–283.

Najavits, L. M., Weiss, R. D., Shaw, S. R., & Muenz, L. R. (1998). "Seeking Safety": Outcome of a new cognitive–behavioral psychotherapy for women with post-traumatic stress disorder and substance dependence. *Journal of Traumatic Stress, 11*, 437–455.

Pennebaker, J. W. (1999). The effects of traumatic disclosure on physical and mental health: The values of writing and talking about upsetting events. *International Journal of Emergency Mental Health, 1*, 9–18.

Polusny, M. A., & Follette, V. M. (1995). Long-term correlates of child sexual abuse: Theory and review of the empirical literature. *Applied and Preventive Psychology, 4*, 143–166.

Resick, P. A., & Schnicke, M. K. (1993). *Cognitive processing therapy for rape victims: A treatment manual.* Newbury Park, CA: Sage.

Resnick, H., Acierno, R., Holmes, M., Dammeyer, M., & Kilpatrick, D. (2000). Emergency evaluation and intervention with female victims of rape and other violence. *Journal of Clinical Psychology, 56,* 1317–1333.

Resnick, H. S., Acierno, R., & Kilpatrick, D. G. (1997). Health impact of interpersonal violence 2: Medical and mental health outcomes. *Behavioral Medicine, 23,* 65–78.

Resnick, H. S., Holmes, M. M., Kilpatrick, D. G., Clum, G., Acierno, R., Best, C. L., & Saunders, B. E. (2000). Predictors of postrape medical care in a national sample of women. *American Journal of Preventive Medicine, 19,* 214–219.

Ruzek, J. I., Polusny, M. A., & Abueg, F. R. (1998). Assessment and treatment of concurrent posttraumatic stress disorder and substance abuse. In V. M. Follette, J. I. Ruzek, & F. R. Aubeg (Eds.), *Cognitive–behavioral therapies for trauma* (pp. 226–255). New York: Guilford Press.

Smith, D. W., Davis, J. L., & Fricker, A. E. (2002). *How is child sexual abuse linked to repeat victimization? Cognitions about risk in women with sexual abuse histories.* Manuscript submitted for publication.

Sommers, M. S., Schafer, J., Zink, T., Hutson, L., & Hillard, P. (2001). Injury patterns in women resulting from sexual assault. *Trauma, Violence, and Abuse, 2,* 240–258.

Triffleman, E., Carroll, K., & Kellogg, S. (1999). Substance dependence posttraumatic stress disorder therapy: An integrated cognitive–behavioral approach. *Journal of Substance Abuse Treatment, 17,* 3–14.

Yehuda, R., Giller, E. L., Southwick, S. M., Lowry, M. T., & Mason, J. W. (1991). Hypothalamic pituitary–adrenal dysfunction in posttraumatic stress disorder. *Biological Psychiatry, 30,* 1031–1048.

Zaslav, M. R. (1994). Psychology of comorbid posttraumatic stress disorder and substance abuse: Lessons from combat veterans. *Journal of Psychoactive Drugs, 26,* 393–400.

11

EFFECTS OF CHILDHOOD ABUSE ON CHILDBEARING AND PERINATAL HEALTH

DEBORAH ISSOKSON

Childhood abuse can have an enormous impact on childbearing. Pregnancy, labor and delivery, breastfeeding, and the postpartum period can all trigger memories of past abuse. Women who are abuse survivors may be more vulnerable to depression and other difficulties, ranging from mild to severe. Sexual abuse survivors are particularly vulnerable because childbearing, by its very nature, has strong connections to sexuality. However, all women who have had abusive or neglectful upbringings in their families of origin may be at risk. This chapter highlights some of the possible areas of difficulty for childbearing abuse survivors and offers specific suggestions for intervention.

The process of bearing a child is one of enormous growth, change, challenge, and stress. It is a normative developmental life crisis that affects every aspect of a woman's life. Vulnerability is inherent in such a transformation. For an abuse survivor, this vulnerability includes the possibility that childbearing will trigger memories of her abuse. For some women, these memories will be familiar and expected. Other women may experience these memories as regressive in their healing process. For still other women, the memories will be unexpected and may signal the first time such memories are coming to the surface. For these women, their childbearing time may be the life event that begins their acknowledgement of their abuse history and thus the beginning of their healing process.

As you work with women, it is probable that you will encounter a client who is both a survivor of abuse and having a baby. If this woman is an acknowledged abuse survivor who has been involved in an active healing process, your task as the provider is threefold: (a) help her maintain her current level of functioning, (b) contain the memories, and (c) facilitate further healing using childbearing as the vehicle for growth.

If this client is not aware of her abuse history, you may suspect an abuse history. According to Courtois and Riley (1992), memories of abuse may be fragmented or absent entirely. They may be recalled only by "triggers," either within the environment or in themselves. The Pandora's box of sexual abuse memories must be opened delicately during the childbearing time. Although, as medical and mental health professionals, we have no control over what lessons a woman will learn during her childbearing experience, we can facilitate a gentle, well-paced, appropriate exploration of issues and history. With all childbearing clients, the ultimate goal is to help the woman have a positive childbearing experience and make a healthy psychological adjustment to motherhood.

This chapter is written primarily for mental health providers working with abuse survivors who are bearing children; however, it is relevant to medical personnel as well. In it, I highlight signals to look for during the childbearing time that might indicate that a woman is an abuse survivor. The chapter is broken down into six sections. The first five address phases of childbearing: (a) pregnancy, (b) labor and delivery, (c) the postpartum period, (d) breastfeeding, (e) infertility and pregnancy loss. In the sixth section I address ways in which mental health providers can work collaboratively with other perinatal care providers and educators.

PREGNANCY

From the moment a pregnancy is confirmed, women begin to create fantasies and images of their babies and themselves as mothers. Ambivalence is inherent, as it is in any undertaking of this magnitude, regardless of how planned and wanted the baby is. What follows is a description of the ways in which an abuse survivor may experience pregnancy.

Physical Experience of Pregnancy

The physical experience of pregnancy can be one of mystery and fascination as well as one of discomfort and sickness. Nausea, vomiting, sore breasts, and weight gain, which often accompany early pregnancy, can cause an abuse survivor to feel out of control of her body very early on. Later in pregnancy, fetal movement can be experienced as intrusive. A woman may cope with these physical challenges of pregnancy by becoming hypervigilant about her body changes and pregnancy symptoms. This hypervigilence, and its accompanying anxiety, can result in a worsening of the symptoms and may be a manifestation of posttraumatic stress disorder (PTSD).

A recent study demonstrated that PTSD can have a negative impact on pregnancy outcomes (Seng et al., 2001). In a large sample of pregnant women, women with PTSD had higher odds ratios of ectopic pregnancy, spontaneous abortion, preterm contractions, hyperemesis, and excessive fetal growth. These findings held even after controlling for possible confounds, including demographic and psychosocial factors.

Women may contact their midwives or obstetricians multiple times between appointments, restrict their diets to avoid weight gain, or dissociate from their growing babies and not allow themselves to bond: experiencing the baby as an intruder and the culprit in her pain and discomfort. They may reject their bodily changes because they are evidence of their sexuality. In addition, they may self-medicate to cope with anxiety. In a study of pregnant women in Norway, sexual abuse survivors were significantly more likely to smoke during pregnancy than their nonabused counterparts (Grimstad & Schei, 1999).

You can encourage women to rely on healthy coping techniques that they have used before. You can also contextualize the changes happening in their bodies and help them adapt to these changes. They may require extensive education on what their bodies are doing, because they may feel alienated or detached from their bodies as a result of the abuse they experienced (Courtois & Riley, 1992). When speaking to a woman, suggest that her body knows exactly what to do to grow this baby. Pregnancy can be a time of enormous healing in terms of a woman reclaiming the wisdom of her body.

Choosing a Perinatal Health Care Provider

To ensure the health and well-being of mother and baby, your client will choose a care provider to follow her throughout the pregnancy and to attend her birth. In a recent qualitative analysis (Seng, Sparbel, Low, & Killion, 2002), researchers found that three groups emerged among childbearing abuse survivors. Members of the first group were far along in their recovery. They had the best childbearing experiences. The type of care that they wanted was that of a collaborative ally—someone with whom they could discuss their concerns and think through ways to make the experience easier. Women in the second group were "not safe"; they sought care from a "compassionate authority figure." Last, members of the third group were not ready to deal with their past but sought a "therapeutic mentor" as a care provider.

I encourage clients to inform their caregivers of their abuse history. Although it is not necessary to tell the entire story, it can be helpful for a provider to have a general sense of the history so that she or he can be sensitized to the client's issues as they pertain to labor and delivery and prenatal and postpartum care. Your client may be dealing with a group practice of providers rather than a single caregiver. This means that she may see a variety of providers over the course of her pregnancy. This also means that the provider attending her birth may be someone she has never met. If she is working with a group practice, she may not want to repeat her story over and over for each provider she encounters. In this case, I advise clients to tell one provider with whom they feel the most comfortable and then ask that a brief note be put in their chart to inform the other providers. A woman can even write a brief statement herself, which can be put in her medical chart. It may also be advisable that you speak with her health care provider during her pregnancy to sensitize her or him to the special needs of this woman given her history.

It is helpful to periodically check in with your client about her relationship with her perinatal care provider. Does she feel respected, heard, and validated? Does she feel safe? Does she have a voice in the relationship? Does she feel there is partnership between herself and the provider in the care of her pregnancy and preparation for birth? You can be instrumental in facilitating her empowerment as she navigates the health care system, all the time encouraging her to trust her instincts as she makes her decisions regarding providers. Given the vulnerability inherent in the childbearing process, a supportive partnership with open communication is crucial for the pregnant abuse survivor.

Choosing a Place to Give Birth

Your client's choice for place of birth may also have a connection to her abuse history. A woman may choose a home birth with a midwife, if she feels most safe and comfortable in her own environment surrounded by family or friends. She may feel that this is the place in which she can have the most control, the place where she can have her voice and best protect herself and her baby. This woman may feel strongly about not having any medical interventions, wanting to be present physically and emotionally for the entire labor and birth experience. She may perceive that there will be pressure in a medical setting to have drugs for the pain. The choice of a home birth will ensure that the same provider will be with her for the entire experience, from the beginning of prenatal care through the postpartum period. Such continuity of care may feel essential for this woman.

On the other end of the continuum is the woman who chooses a hospital birth with a medical doctor. She may perceive this to be the best way for her to take care of herself and her baby; she may feel comfortable in a more passive role by deferring to her doctor, feeling protected by the authority of the hospital. She may feel strongly that it will be healing for her to use drugs for the pain, thus choosing, perhaps for the first time, to say "no" to physical pain.

Prenatal Medical Procedures

For some women, the actual medical procedures that are standard during prenatal care may cause anxiety, trigger memories, or be experienced as intolerable or intrusive. Pelvic examinations, blood pressure checks, and blood draws are the most typical of procedures that cause angst. Some women experience ultrasound as intrusive (J. Kitzinger, 1992). Women may avoid prenatal care altogether so they do not have to go through these procedures (Grant, 1992).

Working with your client on anticipating the procedures, using relaxation and desensitization techniques, and having your client communicate with her provider can help to make these medical procedures less traumatic. If the provider knows of the woman's history, then she or he has a context for the patient's fears and anxieties. This shared knowledge can facilitate a more effective working relationship. You can help your client rehearse good communication so that she is prepared to negotiate the ways in which the difficult medical procedures will be carried out.

Psychological Tasks of Pregnancy

The psychological tasks of pregnancy are universal and yet are always affected by a woman's past and present. For an abuse survivor, the abuse experience brings with it issues unique to each woman's story and her level of healing. The sections that follow comprise an overview of some of these psychological tasks, the accompanying challenges that your client may experience, and suggestions for intervention in the therapy.

Acceptance of Pregnancy

Acceptance of pregnancy is the first psychological task. This includes coming to a place of wanting the pregnancy and the baby, having a positive demeanor during most of the pregnancy, seeking out appropriate health care, being proactive in addressing the discomforts of pregnancy, accepting bodily changes, and allowing for normal ambivalence (Lederman, 1996.)

For an abuse survivor, there may be several challenges in this task. Despite wanting a baby and planning a pregnancy, an abuse survivor may experience doubt early on as to her ability to care for or protect a baby or child. She is all too aware of the dangers of the world and the ways in which adults cannot or do not protect children. In response to her doubts and fears, she may hesitate in embracing the reality of her pregnancy (Grant, 1992). She may ignore her physical changes, dismiss self-care, and postpone prenatal care. Although her doubts and questions about her ability to parent make sense in the context of her history, she may look for any sign that points to the wrongness of her decision to parent.

Depending on your client's level of self-esteem, she may believe that in spite of her wish to parent, she does not deserve to be a parent. She may vacillate between joy and excitement and dread and regret. Ambivalence may be experienced by the survivor as proof that she should not be a parent. You can help your client explore her feelings about her pregnancy. Educate her about the normalcy of ambivalence. Remind her that she has the entire length of the pregnancy to integrate the pregnancy experience. Empower her to set the pace. As will be true with each phase of the childbearing experience, containment of affect, management of memories and flashbacks, and maintenance of a healthy level of functioning remain priorities. As stated earlier, healthy tried-and-true coping strategies work best, with new ones created when necessary.

Relationships With Self and Others

The social aspects and public nature of pregnancy present psychological challenges to the pregnant abuse survivor. Once she starts showing, her pregnancy is clear evidence that she has been sexual (although she may have conceived with the help of reproductive technology). Depending on her relationship to her sexuality, she may feel self-conscious, ashamed, or proud. Although some women want public attention, and even a touch to the belly, others find this intrusive and reminiscent of poor boundaries regarding body integrity and sexuality. If this latter response is the case with your client, you can help her practice different responses she can give to people as a way of setting healthy and safe boundaries for herself.

At some time in her pregnancy, a pregnant woman must begin to see herself as a mother and begin to connect with her growing child. This happens at varying times for each woman and at varying paces. As stated above, an abuse survivor may have fears about being able to adequately protect a child or even that she herself will abuse her child (J. Kitzinger, 1992). These fears can interfere with the developing parental self-concept. From the beginning of pregnancy, a woman who is an abuse survivor may hope for a male child, believing sons are less vulnerable and easier to protect.

On the other hand, she may hope for a female child, with fantasies of correcting her own childhood experience of abuse through parenting a daughter. These gender preferences may complicate her process of bonding with her pregnancy and her baby.

As with all pregnant women, the woman's relationship with her own mother influences the process of maternal identity formation. If your client's mother was not protective or was the perpetrator of abuse, this will be an important time for the abuse survivor to differentiate herself from her mother. Help her explore her notions of what a "good mother" is and encourage her to seek out positive maternal role models.

Your client may struggle with the notion that her perpetrator, and perhaps the person who did not protect her, will be a relative of the baby's, either as a grandparent, aunt, uncle, or cousin. She will need to spend some time sorting out her feelings. She will need to decide whether and how she wants to facilitate a relationship between this person and the baby. If she does choose to cultivate this relationship, she can spend some time in therapy working on setting appropriate boundaries so that she can keep herself safe emotionally and her baby safe physically.

Depression, Anxiety, and Posttraumatic Stress Disorder

Throughout pregnancy, a woman with a history of depression, anxiety, or PTSD is at risk for a recurrence of depression or anxiety (Sichel & Driscoll, 1999). This means that an abuse survivor is at high risk for these difficulties. It is incumbent on you to be vigilant concerning symptoms of mental health problems and to intervene and treat them as soon as possible. Psychotropic medication is an option during pregnancy. Be sure to cultivate relationships with psychopharmacologists who are knowledgeable about treating pregnant and lactating women.

The benefit of the length of pregnancy is that it provides ample opportunity for the pregnant survivor to adjust to the pregnancy and the idea of motherhood. There is time to anticipate the issues that might arise given her history of abuse and to put coping strategies into place. There is time to deal with any issues that arise unexpectedly. Pregnancy can be a time of challenge for survivors of abuse; it can also be a time of great healing.

LABOR AND DELIVERY

Preparation

At some point in pregnancy, a woman must begin to think about labor and delivery. There are many different ways to prepare for birth, and each woman must find that which suits her best. Preparation includes becoming knowledgeable about the process of labor and birth, addressing fears associated with birthing, and ultimately embracing the notion that soon a baby will arrive and that life will permanently change. Although the mechanisms of labor and birth are universal, the ways in which the birthing process unfolds and is experienced is shaped, in part, by a woman's history. For an abuse survivor, the normal fears, anxieties, and concerns about labor and delivery can take on an additional psychic charge due to the physical and sexual nature of birth. On one end of the continuum is the abuse survivor who experiences giving birth as the ultimate healing experience; on the other end is the woman who feels that her birthing experience is tantamount to a recurrence of sexual abuse (J. Kitzinger, 1992; Rhodes & Hutchinson, 1994). There are many levels in between.

Develop Coping Strategies

You will probably not be attending your client's birth as one of her support people; however, you can help her prepare for the birth experience by being aware of the issues that may arise for her. You can help her anticipate the potential triggers for her memories and help her develop a means for staying grounded and present if there is an intrusion of memories or flashbacks (Simkin, 1992). You can help her create strategies for coping with the pain of labor. This is also a time to review healthy coping strategies that she already has in place for dealing with emotional and physical pain. You can encourage her to keep self-care a priority. As part of self-care, empower her to ask for and accept support.

Birth Support

Part of self-care includes lining up appropriate support for the birth. This will probably include her partner (if she has one), and perhaps a friend or other relative with whom she is comfortable. She may want to consider hiring a doula, a professional labor support companion who remains with her for the entirety of the labor and birth process. Studies have shown that the presence of a doula can decrease the length of labor and decrease the need for medical intervention, including pain medication (Klaus, Kennell, & Klaus, 1993). The doula can act as an advocate on behalf of the woman and will ensure continuity of care from at least one birthing professional. Doulas are helpful for all women. For a survivor of sexual abuse, a doula can be her voice if she loses it, her guardian angel so that she does not have to dissociate, and instead can help her stay present for the birth experience. A doula can also support the partner as he or she supports the birthing woman.

Potential Triggers During Labor and Birth

Given the physical and sexual nature of labor and delivery, there is great potential for memories—both body and cognitive memories—to be triggered during the birthing process (Simkin, 1992). For women who are well into their healing process, these triggers can be concretely prepared for, with strategies in place for coping. For women who are unaware of their history, the birthing process may be the launching pad for their first memories of their abuse. It is unfortunate that this situation cannot be prepared for in therapy, but it will need to be processed in therapy during the postpartum period. The following is a brief description of the kinds of stimuli present in the birthing process that can trigger abuse memories and flashbacks. Not all women will respond in the same way to these stimuli, but it will be helpful for you to keep this list in mind as you help your client prepare realistically for birth.

The physicality of the labor and delivery speaks for itself. In an ethnographic study of labor and delivery (Rhodes & Hutchinson, 1994), a number of potential triggers were identified. These included nakedness, vaginal exams, and pain in the pelvic and genital areas of the body, blood and other bodily secretions, body odors, changes in breathing, crying, and moaning. Labor involves exposure of body parts to other people, many of whom are in positions of authority, some of whom are even strangers.

Labor and birth take on a life of their own, often feeling out of control to the birthing woman. Although a woman can say "no" to the pain and ask for medication, she cannot say "no" to the birth process; she must complete it. A woman may fear pain medication or anesthesia because she is afraid of being numbed out from the physical sensations of birth, and she feels less in control and more vulnerable. In response to the physical experience of birthing, some abuse survivors will perceive the process similar to rape. Some women will fear their bodies are being mutilated. Some women fear they are dying. The baby moving through the vagina can be experienced as forced penetration. Many abuse survivors will use dissociation as a coping strategy. Other coping styles include passivity, belligerence, and counterdependence. Some women may experience anxiety attacks. Others will become controlling and uncooperative with caregivers (Rhodes & Hutchinson, 1994).

Again, the presence of a doula can be invaluable during these times. A doula typically has spent some time getting to know the woman prior to the birth and has had time to develop a trusting relationship with her. You may even include the doula in a therapy session to ensure good communication and to answer any questions the doula may have about helping the birthing woman to stay grounded and present during the birthing process. Because a doula is trained and has attended many births, she is in a good position to help the woman anticipate the process and to pace herself through it emotionally. Depending on your client's issues with trust, she may need to do some work regarding being able to trust that her entire birth team can keep her safe during this vulnerable experience and will do everything possible to protect her from harm. Again, the goal is to help the woman contain her memories, to continue functioning in a healthy manner throughout the process of birth and into the postpartum period, and to facilitate further growth.

Although most births have healthy and uncomplicated physical outcomes, the emotional outcome is not so predictable. Despite great preparation and anticipatory work, there is no way to know how a woman will experience the psychic process of birthing. There is no way to know ahead of time what life lessons she will learn, what historical issues will be stirred up, and how she will make meaning of this experience. Although her partner, doula, or other health care providers may perceive the birth to have been wonderful, empowering, and successful, the woman herself may have a completely different emotional experience and perception of the same event. Furthermore, the emotional outcome is an unfolding process for the postpartum woman. As I discuss in the next section, the new mother spends a part of her postpartum time reviewing and dissecting her birthing experience. It is not unusual for the survivor of abuse, years later, to have a new perspective on her experience. Sometimes it is a more healing perspective; other times, it is a perspective that now includes a deeper understanding of and connection to the relationship between her abuse history and her birthing experience.

THE POSTPARTUM PERIOD

Adjustment to Parenting

The postpartum period consists of the first year after the birth of a baby. For an abuse survivor, the postpartum period can be a time of consolidation of past healing efforts as she enters a phase of parenting and protecting a new human being. For other survivors, parenting can be the catalyst for new memories and flashbacks, new conflicts with extended family, and even regression in the healing process. The following is a description of some particular issues that may arise for abuse survivors who are new mothers.

Mother–Infant Bonding

Just as the pregnant survivor questions her ability to mother and protect her baby, so too will the postpartum survivor. Depending on her level of self-esteem and her identification as a victim, she may question whether she has anything to offer to her baby. Some women will have difficulties bonding with their babies. This difficulty may be related to the gender of the baby or whom the baby physically resembles. In response to the baby's constant needs and demands, the mother may project adult characteristics onto the baby and see the baby as a perpetrator, always needing something from her, always wanting physical contact, not knowing any boundaries. The new mother may fear hurting her baby and perpetrating abuse herself. She may feel angry and frustrated with a crying or inconsolable baby (S. Kitzinger, 1990). The mother might question the appropriateness of touching the baby's genitals as she changes or washes the baby. She may feel frightened to be left alone with the baby. All new mothers reflect on their own experience of being mothered. For an abuse survivor who was not protected by her mother, or for a woman whose perpetrator may have been her own mother or a mother figure, new motherhood may raise new feelings, memories, flashbacks, and fears that will need to be processed and worked out in the therapy.

Maternal Identity Formation

Just as it was helpful during pregnancy to encourage your client to seek out good mothering role models, it continues to be helpful in the postpartum period. Encourage your client to take an inventory of her talents, skills, values, and strengths that she brings to bear on mothering. Remind her that she does not need to know how to do it all right now. Mothering is a process, and the mother–child relationship is one into which she will grow over time. She can set the pace. Give her permission to feel vulnerable and clumsy. It is vital that she seek out postpartum support groups for peer support. There may be a specific group for new mothers who are abuse survivors. She may feel most comfortable in a group of women with this shared history. You may even decide to start such a group yourself. If there is no such group available, keep in mind that your client will have much in common with all new mothers, and, in fact, being in a general postpartum group may help her to normalize her feelings and experiences, thus feeling more connected to the general population of new mothers (Kendall-Tackett, 2001).

Family Relationships and Boundaries

Abuse survivors often need to revisit the issue of family boundaries regarding relationships with family members who may have been part of the abuse history. Boundaries previously set may need to be reworked, and new boundaries may need to be put in place to ensure the baby's safety. If a mother is clear that she does not want certain extended family members to have contact with the baby, then she may need to grieve any fantasies she may have held of the kind of relationships she would have wished for her baby to have with extended family. This may mean not having a relationship with grandparents or uncles or cousins.

Integration of the Birth Experience

All women review and integrate their birth experience over time. If your client had a satisfying experience, you can use her reflections on her birth experience as a catalyst for further growth regarding strength, empowerment, ability to rise to challenges, trust in self and body, and ability to take risks. If your client had a dissatisfying or traumatic birth experience, your task is to help her process the experience, grieve her disappointments, and learn from it. You may need to encourage her to talk with her health care providers or members of her birth support team. You may need to help her differentiate between disappointment in herself and disappointment and anger at her caregivers, keeping in mind the possibility of her projections onto her caregivers. The integration of the birth experience takes time, and it may not happen right away. Your client will reflect on her birth experience for a long time to come.

Postpartum Mental Health

Risk factors for postpartum mental health problems include a previous history of depression or anxiety, history of abuse, relationship problems, social isolation, traumatic birth experience, and health problems in the mother or baby (Buist, 1998). Survivors of abuse are at high risk for experiencing postpartum depressive and anxiety disorders. A recent study of women who suffered from major depression during the postpartum period indicated that 50% of them were sexual abuse survivors. The sexually abused women had higher depression and anxiety scores and less improvement over time—even when compared with other depressed women (Buist & Janson, 2001).

These are mental health issues that require attention and treatment as soon as possible, as they have a detrimental impact not only on the woman but also on her baby and her entire family. Postpartum depression and postpartum anxiety can occur at any point during the postpartum year. Studies indicate that 10% to 20% of new mothers will experience one of these disorders. One in 1,000 will experience postpartum psychosis, which requires immediate hospitalization and medication (Sichel & Driscoll, 1999).

It is important not to underestimate the impact of the stresses of new motherhood on mood and mental health. Shame may keep a new mother from disclosing how miserable or overwhelmed she feels. Early detection and intervention can change the course of family functioning. Postpartum mood disorders are treatable.

All new mothers need to be mothered themselves. As they make this transition to motherhood, they need support, both practical and emotional. This help can come from relatives, friends, or hired help. It may come from support groups, home visiting resources, and on-line chat rooms. You will do your client a great service by encouraging and promoting these networks of support, even suggesting that your client arrange for them before giving birth. They are vital to a new mother's well-being. Anticipatory work and preventive interventions during the prenatal period are ideal. However, if you do not begin working with your client until after she has given birth, understand that it is never too late to provide postpartum support and resources. Interventions on behalf of the mother benefit the baby and the entire family system.

BREASTFEEDING

Breastfeeding a baby is part of the ideal vision of mothering for many women. Many care providers assume that abuse survivors do not want to breastfeed. However, two studies have found that a significantly higher percentage of women planned to breastfeed (Benedict, Paine, & Paine, 1994) and initiated breastfeeding after birth (Prentice, Lu, Lange, & Halfon, 2002).

Even when women want to breastfeed, there are aspects of this experience that can prove difficult. Common challenges in the early weeks of breastfeeding include sore nipples, positioning difficulties, and milk supply concerns. For abuse survivors, the challenges can multiply. The physical contact at the breast may trigger flashbacks; these reactions and emotions may be intensified if breastfeeding is painful. A lactation consultant or breastfeeding peer counselor may be helpful in establishing a solid breastfeeding relationship. However, an abuse survivor may feel inhibited and uncomfortable having strangers touching her breasts or putting the baby to her breast in an attempt to teach good positioning. A lactation consultant may also be able to help the mother talk through her discomforts and concerns, thus reframing the breastfeeding experience in a way that makes it tolerable for the mother.

Some women feel confused about the dual function of their breasts as both the source of nutrition for their babies and a source of sexual pleasure for themselves and their partners. They may feel ashamed and dumbfounded if they experience any feelings of arousal during breastfeeding, although that is completely normal. A woman may feel uncomfortable if her baby interacts playfully with her breasts during feedings (Kendall-Tackett, 1998).

Breastfeeding in public may feel awkward, inappropriate, exhibitionistic, or immodest. A lactation consultant can show your client techniques for discreet breastfeeding, especially if she is concerned about being exposed in public or at home. Encourage attendance at La Leche League meetings or other breastfeeding support groups (hospitals often have these). At these gatherings, your client will see the ways in which other new mothers manage public breastfeeding, they will have breastfeeding normalized for them, and they will be in a safe place to talk about the breastfeeding experience.

Breast pumps are a common tool to aid in breastfeeding. They are used for mothers who have premature or hospitalized babies and need to maintain their milk supply. They can be used for mothers who plan to return to work after the baby is born, or they can be used for mothers who find it intolerable to put their babies to breast but want to provide breast milk. Some women find the breast pump painful, particularly if they are using a small, battery-operated pump. For mothers who need to pump on a regular basis, the electric hospital-grade pumps are a better choice. These are more comfortable and more efficient in removing milk from the breast. However, even with these, some women feel that it objectifies their breasts and makes them feel like a "milking machine." The tugging and pulling at the breast can be hard for abuse survivors to tolerate. Other abuse survivors find it freeing because it allows alternative methods of feeding, and it allows for someone else to feed the baby. This is a huge relief for many women as it ensures the baby receives breast milk while at the same time giving the mother some space and time for herself.

As mentioned in the beginning of this section, for many women the breastfeeding relationship is the quintessential vision of early mothering. As such, there is great emphasis on successful and satisfying breastfeeding. For all women, and in this case for abuse survivors, the temptation to cease breastfeeding in the face of physical, social, and emotional difficulties is fraught with conflict. If a woman decides to stop breastfeeding because of difficulties, she is often racked by guilt and shame. If she continues with stoicism and pain, she may dissociate during breastfeeding or become resentful toward her baby. With the help of a lactation consultant, the woman may be able to come up with a plan for modified breastfeeding without pain, augmented by alternative methods of feeding. If the breastfeeding experience proves to be too emotionally laden, then give your client permission to use an alternate feeding method. Ultimately, it is most important that she be emotionally available to her baby, and if alternate methods of feeding will facilitate this bonding, then that is the priority.

As a therapist, you can support your client's breastfeeding intentions and efforts and at the same time assist her in making healthy decisions for herself and her relationship with her baby. This may entail some work concerning setting limits and boundaries so that she is not providing mothering at her own emotional expense. With your client's permission, it may be helpful for you to speak with the breastfeeding support person so that you can ensure that you are both in sync with the feeding plan. The early feeding experience is often very important for a new mother. The idea that she may not be able to nourish her baby sufficiently can be emotionally devastating. Conversely, mothers who see their babies plump up before their very eyes beam a level of satisfaction and pride that is beyond words (Kendall-Tackett, 1998, 2001).

INFERTILITY AND PREGNANCY LOSS

For many women, the ability to conceive and carry a pregnancy to term is a milestone in terms of securing a sense of confidence in their bodies. Women who are abuse survivors may already have a conflictual relationship with their bodies and their sexuality. They may question the functioning and adequacy of their bodies. Difficulty either in conceiving or in carrying a pregnancy to term can trigger issues of body betrayal and failure as a woman and as a sexual being.

Infertility diagnosis and treatment involves many invasive procedures over a prolonged period of time. It involves reliance on medical personnel who are often given great authority over a woman's reproductive fate. This is a challenge for any woman. Superimpose issues common to abuse survivors, and the process of conceiving a child through reproductive technology is not only stressful but also ripe for triggering memories of abuse and symptoms of PTSD.

There are several ways to be helpful to a client who is struggling with any form of infertility, including pregnancy loss. First, be sure that your client uses stress management and relaxation techniques. Infertility is stressful psychologically, interpersonally, sexually, and physically. Relationships often suffer during infertility treatment as well as during decision making concerning ongoing treatment or the cessation of treatment. Sexual intimacy is often scheduled, regardless of desire. The treatments, particularly the hormonal drug treatments, can wreak havoc on a woman's mood and lability. Psychologically, she is often in a state of limbo, waiting for a menstrual period, waiting to begin a cycle of drugs, waiting for a positive pregnancy test or a call from a clinic about the viability of embryos. Encourage participation in a peer support group. Be available to discuss fears, anxieties, goals, and thresholds for treatment. When appropriate, help her make connections between her current challenges and her abuse history and, as always, use this context as a vehicle for further healing.

COLLABORATIVE CARE

To provide comprehensive care to women during their childbearing time, you must have an adequate understanding not only of the psychological and developmental processes a woman undergoes but also of the physiological processes and medical procedures that are part and parcel of pregnancy, birth, and the postpartum period. This is particularly important when working with survivors of abuse who are pregnant, for we know that the sequelae of sexual abuse can have a far-reaching impact not only on mental health but also on physical and sexual health (Moeller, Bachmann, & Moeller, 1993). A multidisciplinary approach to the provision of care for childbearing women—one in which mental health providers work alongside obstetrical providers—is ideal. However, because these arrangements are few and far between, you can consider developing a collaborative relationship with health care and childbirth professionals in your community (Seng & Hassinger, 1998).

The following is a list of the various professionals a pregnant or post-partum woman might encounter: midwife, obstetrician or family practitioner, childbirth educator, nutritionist, doula (professional labor support companion), postpartum doula, breastfeeding counselor, lactation consultant, baby nurse, and pediatrician. Create a working relationship with these providers in your community as well as with a psychopharmacologist in your area who is knowledgeable about medications used during pregnancy and lactation. These colleagues will be a vital resource to you and your clients. For women whose lives were chaotic because of the abuse, and for women who have concerns that their issues are "too big" for any one provider, collaborative care on their behalf can feel comforting (Seng & Hassinger, 1998). They feel protected, as if all their bases will be covered. Collaborating with colleagues during this time of heightened vulnerability for your client can be relieving for you as well. It allows you to share the responsibility of facilitating a positive childbearing experience for your client and ensuring her healthy adjustment to motherhood. It models for her the act of reaching out for help and creating a community of support, which is ultimately what she needs to do for herself and her growing family.

In addition to cultivating relationships with other perinatal service providers, you may find it useful to refer to books, Web sites, and organizations that address the needs of childbearing women and their families. For a comprehensive list of resources, visit http://www.reproheart.com, click on Health Professionals, and select Resource List for Book Chapter *Effects of Childhood Abuse on Childbearing and Perinatal Health*. See the end of this chapter for a brief list of resources to get you started.

CONCLUSION

Throughout this chapter, I have emphasized the importance of helping your childbearing client contain her abuse memories, maintain a healthy level of functioning, and further her healing and growth in the context of her childbearing experience. This happens as you explore together the connections between her abuse history and the issues that arise for her during pregnancy, birth, and the postpartum period. Her task is to make meaning of her symptoms, her feelings, and her experience. Let her set the pace for this exploration. When working with a client who has already completed a fair amount of healing work, remind her that a recurrence of PTSD symptoms is not necessarily a sign of regression; rather, it is an indication that this new experience of childbearing is touching on some new or unexplored aspects of her history that she did not have to previously confront. With the client who has had little or no knowledge of having been abused, move gently with her as she explores her associations and concerns during childbearing, and allow her to make her own connections to her history at her own pace.

Empower your client to shape this childbearing experience for herself. Anticipate potential triggers. Remind her of her existent coping strategies. Help her create a safe and egalitarian working relationship with her health care provider. Encourage her to gather a support network of family, friends, and professionals who can assist her in her journey into motherhood. Your work together ideally can culminate in a positive emotional experience of pregnancy and birth, a healthy connection between mother and baby, and the client's sense of self-efficacy as a mother.

ADDITIONAL RESOURCES

Pregnancy: http://www.parentsplace.com/pregnancy
Doulas: http://www.dona.org
Postpartum depression: http://depressionafterdeliver.com
Breastfeeding: http://www.lalecheleague.org
Perinatal loss: http://www.hygeia.org
Infertility: http://www.resolve.org
Abortion: http://www.afterabortion.org

REFERENCES

Benedict, M., Paine, L., & Paine, L. (1994). *Long-term effects of child sexual abuse on functioning in pregnancy and pregnancy outcome* (Final report, National Center on Child Abuse and Neglect). Washington, DC: National Center on Child Abuse and Neglect.

Buist, A. (1998). Childhood abuse, postpartum depression and parenting difficulties: A literature review of associations. *Australian and New Zealand Journal of Psychiatry, 32*, 370–378.

Buist, A., & Janson, H. (2001). Childhood sexual abuse, parenting, and postpartum depression: A 3-year follow-up study. *Child Abuse and Neglect, 25*, 909–921.

Courtois, C. A., & Riley, C. C. (1992). Pregnancy and childbirth as triggers for abuse memories: Implications for care. *Birth, 19*, 222–223.

Grant, L. J. (1992). Effects of childhood sexual abuse: Issues for obstetric caregivers. *Birth, 19*, 220–221.

Grimstad, H., & Schei, B. (1999). Pregnancy and delivery for women with a history of child sexual abuse. *Child Abuse and Neglect, 23*, 81–90.

Kendall-Tackett, K. A. (1998). Breastfeeding and the sexual abuse survivor. *Journal of Human Lactation, 14*, 125–130.

Kendall-Tackett, K. A. (2001). *The hidden feelings of motherhood: Coping with stress, depression and burnout.* Oakland, CA: New Harbinger.

Kitzinger, J. (1992). Counteracting, not reenacting, the violation of women's bodies: The challenge for perinatal caregivers. *Birth, 19*, 219–221.

Kitzinger, S. (1990). *The crying baby.* New York: Penguin.

Klaus, M. H., Kennell, J. H., & Klaus, P. H. (1993). *Mothering the mother.* Reading, MA: Addison-Wesley.

Lederman, R. P. (1996). *Psychosocial adaptation to pregnancy* (2nd ed.). New York: Springer.

Moeller, T. P., Bachmann, G. A., & Moeller, J. R. (1993). The combined effects of physical, sexual, and emotional abuse during childhood: Long-term health consequences for women. *Child Abuse & Neglect, 17*, 623–640.

Prentice, J. C., Lu, M. C., Lange, L., & Halfon, N. (2002). The association between reported childhood sexual abuse and breastfeeding initiation. *Journal of Human Lactation, 18*, 219–226.

Rhodes, N., & Hutchinson, S. (1994). Labor experiences of childhood sexual abuse survivors. *Birth, 21*, 213–220.

Seng, J. S., & Hassinger, J. A. (1998). Improving maternity care with survivors of childhood sexual abuse. *Journal of Nurse-Midwifery, 43*, 287–295.

Seng, J. S., Oakley, D. J., Sampselle, C. M., Killion, C., Graham-Bermann, S., & Liberzon, I. (2001). Posttraumatic stress disorder and pregnancy complications. *Obstetrics and Gynecology, 97*, 17–22.

Seng, J. S., Sparbel, K. J., Low, L. K., & Killion, C. (2002). Abuse-related posttraumatic stress and desired maternity care practices: Women's perspectives. *Journal of Midwifery and Women's Health, 47*, 360–370.

Sichel, D., & Driscoll, J. W. (1999). *Women's moods: What every woman must know about hormones, the brain, and emotional health.* New York: Morrow.

Simkin, P. (1992). Overcoming the legacy of childhood sexual abuse: The role of caregivers and childbirth educators. *Birth, 19*, 224–225.

12

MINDING THE BODY: THE INTERSECTION OF DISSOCIATION AND PHYSICAL HEALTH IN RELATIONAL TRAUMA PSYCHOTHERAPY

TERRI J. HAVEN AND LAURIE ANNE PEARLMAN

Dissociation, a hallmark of posttraumatic symptomatology, is often considered a mental health symptom, but dissociation has an impact on physical health as well. This chapter addresses (a) the complex ways in which prolonged dissociation may affect a survivor's physical health and (b) the complexities, challenges, and critical importance of considering physical health within the psychotherapy process with highly dissociative clients. The ideas presented in this chapter reflect a theoretical framework of constructivist self development theory coupled with the authors' own clinical experiences and consultations.

The authors would like to thank Julie Fenster, MS, MPH, for her generous assistance in gathering and organizing the background literature for this chapter. We are also grateful to Eileen P. Drumm, Christine Farber, PhD, Jeanne Folks, DMin, Lynn Matteson, PsyD, Karen Seltzer, MSW, Beth Tabor Lev, PhD, Pamela Taylor, PsyD, and Sally Van Wright, MSW for their helpful comments on drafts of this chapter.

Jane, a 37-year-old professional woman, first entered therapy shortly after the death of her abusive stepfather with the stated goal of "Maybe now I can finally put everything he did behind me." Her body first entered the therapy dialogue through self-harm. As Jane began to talk in therapy about the abuse and torture she had suffered, she began to cut and burn her body frequently. She would often come to session full of shame and self-loathing, unable to find language for how and why her body had new injuries, feeling estranged from herself and from the therapy relationship and able to tell her story only through flashbacks, fragmented memories, and re-enactments. At times, the therapist felt like a helpless witness to Jane's internal conflict of feeling both increasingly young and vulnerable and experiencing a profound self-hatred and the need to punish herself for betraying family secrets. The awareness of this inner struggle helped the therapist to understand that Jane may have originally developed these strategies to maintain her belief that her family loved her and that she deserved the abuse.

The therapist became aware of split-off aspects of Jane's experience of her body through her own maternal countertransference and intense concern for Jane's physical wounds, even though Jane seemed to experience no physical pain from the injuries. Jane described the cutting and burning as bringing her calm, reducing her anxiety, and providing a way of experiencing control and competence. Jane's childhood and early adult experiences with medical providers had been very negative, and thus Jane had met her psychological need for safety by seeking no medical care for the past 10 years. Instead, Jane became very focused on and skilled at self-care of injuries and medical needs of "the body."

With affect ranging from childlike terror to complete numbness, Jane recounted a childhood of severe physical and sexual abuse within her family. These dissociated memories came in a variety of ways: as visual imagery, as sensory memories, as childlike descriptions of body parts, and as the reliving of particularly violent events through nightmares and flashbacks. At times, Jane had difficulty breathing, experienced nausea, and expressed an array of physical aches and pain. At other times, she was unaware of, or seemed numb to, these body symptoms while processing the same event. Much of the therapy centered on helping Jane to develop healthier ways to self-soothe and to distinguish between the past and present.

Jane's horrific stories and re-enactments challenged the therapist to hold her own powerful feelings of horror; sadness; helplessness; rage; fear; the need to disbelieve; and a desire to rescue the small, injured child. All of these feelings were framed within a deep respect and admiration for Jane's courage and ability to survive. Understanding the complexities and necessarily slow pace of this process, the therapist felt moments of dread, both for herself and for Jane, of the pain she knew would continue as Jane remembered, talked, and mourned. As she reflected on her feelings of dread, the therapist then felt shame for her own self-protective need to disconnect and, in a sense, dissociate from the enormity of it all. Consultation and support from colleagues allowed the therapist to remain aware of the context of her own internal dissociative responses and to gain an even deeper appreciation for the adaptive origins of Jane's internal fragmentation.

During the most difficult times of Jane's remembering, the therapist remained connected and relationally present in the work, in part, by focusing on her understanding that "the worst has already happened." Jane's frequent reliving of the events in a childlike state was more tolerable if the therapist viewed the trauma as all in the past and Jane's symptoms as part of her psychological adaptation to that trauma. Unfortunately, this frame of reference limited the consideration of the condition of Jane's body other than that related to self-harm. A medical crisis brought this omission to the forefront of the work.

The therapy session had focused on Jane's deepening connection with sadness and loss related to her experience as an adolescent of a forced abortion of a pregnancy resulting from incest. This mourning process had been a frequent focal point over the past year and, although extremely painful, had begun to help Jane experience herself as less toxic and to connect with her strength as a nurturing mother of her teenage daughter. Often during the processing of the abortion, Jane would state with tears, "My heart hurts." The therapist understood and responded to this statement as an expression of loss, a sense of heartbreak. Within a psychological trauma framework, she did not connect Jane's fluctuating experiences of shortness of breath, nausea, arm pain, and numbness with the "heartache" as a potential physical health problem needing attention. Instead, the therapist had remained joined with Jane in experiencing her body in fragmented, psychological ways. Jane's view of the world as "a place to hide from" and her disconnection from bodily experiences kept her from considering the possibility of seeking help until the pain was unbearable and assistance absolutely unavoidable. Later in the day of this session, Jane was admitted to the hospital for an emergency procedure on her heart.

This therapy is similar to many relational trauma therapies in which dissociation is the underlying psychological defense—a powerful process of longing to connect and needing to disconnect—of not knowing, not noticing, not remembering. To do the work, both Jane and her therapist needed to subscribe to the belief that "at least there is no more pain." Relational trauma therapists are asked to hold an incredible amount of affect for themselves and their clients, often for years, as clients integrate their histories and the consequences.

We could certainly reflect on the "what if" about this phase of the therapy with Jane. What if the therapist had connected the physical symptoms earlier in the therapy? Would Jane have been able to respond in a way that would have allowed her to seek medical attention before her body was in crisis? How might the therapy relationship have shifted with the inclusion of a discussion of physical health? Would they have found a physician to work in concert with the therapy and with Jane's fragmented understanding of her body? Would Jane's disconnection from her body and her high tolerance for pain make her symptoms seem minimal and therefore misdiagnosed or rejected?

The answers to these questions are unique to the therapy with Jane. However, the overall answer is very clear: Our understanding of and response to psychological adaptations and survival strategies are only part of the treatment picture. For the healing process to be more fully restorative for our trauma survivor clients, we must be willing to widen our lens to assist our clients in being in relationship with their physical bodies—to knowing, to noticing, to feeling, that Jane's heartache was both psychological and physical.

TRAUMA, THE BODY, AND DISSOCIATION: A RELATIONAL APPROACH

Background

Child maltreatment often includes abuse of children's bodies. Despite this reality, and the fact that client and therapist sit together for many hours discussing intimate topics, it is not common for psychotherapies outside of medical settings to include discussion of the client's body or physical health. Therapists and clients can work together for years without talking about the ways in which the abuse the client experienced affected his or her body then and how it continues to affect his or her body now. Despite widespread documentation of the extensive and severe physical health effects of child maltreatment, many complex trauma survivors—people whose symptoms go beyond those of posttraumatic stress disorder (PTSD)—live without medical care, silently experiencing intense and prolonged pain. They may endure unhelpful medical procedures and treatments, suffer more than they would with adequate care, and die prematurely (Felitti et al., 1998). Many of these survivors are receiving regular attention from psychotherapists who are unaware of this central aspect of their clients' experience.

The purpose of this chapter is to expand the frame of psychotherapy with survivors of childhood maltreatment to include attention to the client's physical health. We provide a theoretical framework for understanding the role of dissociation in limiting therapist and client awareness and discussion of physical health, describe a relational approach to working with trauma survivors on physical health issues, and make treatment recommendations based on this conceptualization.

Our approach to working with adults who have experienced severe childhood trauma is based in constructivist self development theory (McCann & Pearlman, 1990; Pearlman & Saakvitne, 1995) and the Risking Connection model (Saakvitne, Gamble, Pearlman, & Lev, 2000). Central to this approach are noticing and naming interpersonal processes in the therapy relationship, including dissociative processes and re-enactments, and naming what is being left out (e.g., in Jane's case, the client's physical health and relationship with her body and health). This approach implies that therapists take an active role in trying to remain aware of and understand with the client the origins and meanings of the client's self-protective psychological processes, including dissociation. At the same time, the therapist must also acknowledge and discuss with the client the very real physical consequences of the physical assault that are central to sexual and other physical abuse.

Psychotherapists may not be aware that something crucial is being left out of the therapy, out of therapist and client awareness, for some very good reasons. Many therapy paradigms, including those developed specifically to treat trauma survivors, address only issues that are part of the classic trauma symptom picture of PTSD, that is, avoidance of reminders of traumatic experiences, intrusion of elements of those experiences, and physiological hyperarousal. That avoidance, which is integral to PTSD, may also be a contributing factor to the lack of conversation about physical health. Only psychodynamic and relational therapies explicitly address the therapeutic relationship, that is, what the therapist and client notice about what is happening between them. Also, the removed stance of a traditional nonrelational psychoanalytic therapist may well reinforce the client's disconnection from her physical experience, despite Freud's emphasis on the body as the center of psychological experiences (Pearlman & Saakvitne, 1995).

Therapists and Physical Health Concerns

Most therapists are not trained to inquire about clients' physical health. We are trained to notice symptoms that fit into areas within which we can assist. So, when a client complains of shortness of breath, gastric discomfort, or muscular aches and pains, we naturally think of anxiety or stress. We may think of somatization. We know how to help with these issues. The essential dualism of much Western healing also invites a disconnection of body, mind, and spirit; if the client doesn't mention his or her body, it's easy for the therapist not to notice or think of it.

What if, in addition to intrapsychic conflict, anxiety, or stress, we thought, "I wonder how my client's body was affected by what she endured in childhood. I wonder whether she might have a physical illness or injury?" Raising such a question could have different meanings, depending on variables such as the client's particular experiences, the nature of the therapeutic relationship, and the timing within the therapy. The client might experience the therapist's inquiry as being seen, being found out. Shame, fear, and a sense of badness are possible responses. Or the client might feel cared for and nurtured. Many survivors don't recognize signs of physical need or distress until the pain is unbearable (Nijenhuis, Vanderlinden, & Spinhoven, 1998) and, therefore, could be confused or surprised by the therapist's question.

If the therapist and client were engaged in a relational therapy that could weather and process these complex feelings, the therapist might then want to work together with the client to consult with a physician. This, too, can bring a range of responses specific to the client and the therapy relationship. Many trauma survivors are very reluctant to seek medical treatment. They may have had traumatic medical-related experiences as children (e.g., "I'll take you to the doctor" is a common threat used to frighten a child). Or children may have had unnecessary procedures or treatments. Many abused children do not receive medical treatment for injuries from repeated abuse. As adults, they may not only have serious physical problems but also may continue to deny themselves medical care, sometimes feeling not entitled or accustomed to care (Saakvitne et al., 2000).

Survivors may have had traumatic encounters with physical health care providers as adults. For example, unaware or insensitive medical providers may have proceeded without introducing themselves or explaining what they were about to do and why. Providers may have had no appreciation of the meanings of physical touch to abuse survivors. When survivors have sought help, they may have experienced repeated unhelpful diagnoses and treatments, or they may have been told, "It's all in your head" or "There's nothing wrong with you." Many survivors feel powerless in relationships with authority figures and unable to advocate for themselves or actively participate in medical appointments (e.g., choosing or changing physicians, asking questions or taking notes during appointments). They may have no health insurance or be unable to pay for health care. The abuse may have created great sensitivities, resulting in shame and fear about their bodies, making medical attention too threatening to contemplate. Changes in religious or spiritual beliefs after traumatic experiences leave some survivors without a sense of faith or meaning and may contribute to the belief that seeking medical care is hopeless. Finally, there may be cultural prohibitions about acknowledging physical illness or seeking treatment (Laria & Lewis-Fernandez, 2001). We are interested in bringing clinicians' attention to the impact of abuse on people's bodies and the long-term direct consequences of that damage. When small children's bodies are abused, any and all of their bodily systems can be affected. These effects can result in long-term physical health consequences beyond somatization, including life-altering physical adaptations and life-threatening illnesses (Felitti et al., 1998; Schnurr, Spiro, & Paris, 2000). How can psychotherapists assist the complex trauma survivor in noticing, naming, and attending to these problems?

Relational Trauma Psychotherapy

Writers at the Stone Center (Jordan, Kaplan, Miller, Stiver, & Surrey, 1991) have defined *relational psychotherapy* as a model of working with clients based on themes of respect, mutuality, and client empowerment. The Stone Center model suggests that "relationship, based on empathic attunement, is the key to the process of therapy, not just the backdrop for it" (Jordan et al., 1991, p. 284). Saakvitne and colleagues (2000) applied the relational model to work with complex trauma survivors in the Risking Connection trauma-training curriculum.

Interwoven in a relational trauma framework is the ongoing process of psychoeducation, generally thought of as including common sources and manifestations of traumatic stress, strategies for managing symptoms, and so on (Saakvitne et al., 2000). However, psychoeducation also provides an important context for naming and normalizing the physical consequences of abuse. Jane's therapist might have provided information as follows:

> We've talked about some of the feelings and responses different people have related to their trauma experience. Many trauma survivors also have physical problems from lack of preventive care during childhood, untreated injuries from abuse, and struggles getting medical care as an adult. We'll work together to understand your experience.

Relational trauma therapy provides the essential opportunity for survivors of childhood abuse and neglect to repair attachment wounds in relationships (Pearlman & Courtois, in press). The therapist's role is to create an environment in which the client can discuss anything that might be affected by childhood maltreatment. That includes areas of the self, such as self-worth, identity, worldview, psychological needs, spirituality, sexuality, and physical health (McCann & Pearlman, 1990; Saakvitne et al., 2000). Although most therapists who work from this perspective allow the client to take the lead in introducing topics for exploration, it is the therapist's responsibility to encourage and sometimes introduce issues where shame, fear, dissociation, or worldview may inhibit the client from doing so. Shame, fear, or dissociation could inhibit the client from bringing in issues related to his or her body, including sexuality and physical health. Worldview may inhibit a client from bringing up anything about which "nothing can be done." One exchange between Jane and her therapist might have gone as follows:

Therapist: You've shared many ways you were violated and hurt as a child. I often find myself wondering how your physical health might be affected now by what happened back then. I don't recall you ever mentioning your health.

Jane: No need to talk about it. I learned a long time ago that I was safer taking care of that myself.

Therapist: For you, safety has meant having to do things alone and hiding your needs. I'd like to work with you to find more ways for you to feel safe. I can imagine what it must be like to work so hard at hiding—even from your own body.

Many complex trauma survivor clients have a great capacity for using dissociation to tolerate both physical and emotional pain, and they experience the great costs of that tolerance. Not feeling something as it is happening, however, does not protect the individual from suffering. Research on peritraumatic dissociation suggests the opposite: People who dissociate at the time of traumatic experiences are at greater risk for later psychological difficulties (see Allen, 2001, for a brief review of the literature on peritraumatic dissociation). Certainly, being out of touch with one's feelings makes it impossible to use feelings as a source of information that would allow self-protection.

When the body is left out of psychotherapies with trauma survivors, a re-enactment is taking place. The body again is a source of shame, the repository for a terrible secret. Goodwin and Attias (1999) and others have noted that one's identity is located in one's body, so if the body must be hidden, then so too must the self. This is an old, familiar story for children whose lives were ruled by fear, including fear of being seen and fear of their needs and feelings. Adult survivors know very well how to keep their needs, feelings, bodily experiences, and shame out of a relationship. Dissociation is a central process in survival for many children who are being abused (Putnam, 1997). They find ways not to know, or not to know everything at once and to compartmentalize their experience to avoid being overwhelmed by it. This process, carried into and not addressed in psychotherapy, of course restricts the gains that can be made.

That is not to say that people's bodies aren't mentioned in trauma therapies. Many complex trauma survivors struggle with self-harming behaviors (Briere & Gil, 1998; Connors, 2000; Miller, 1994; Nicholls, Deiter, & Pearlman, 2000; Santa Mina & Gallop, 1998; Zlotnick et al., 1996). When clients harm themselves, relational therapists may name the damage that cutting or drinking or other self-harming behaviors do to the client's body, and they work with the client to understand what purpose the harm is serving. We pay a great deal of attention to clients' nonverbal behaviors, such as tears, eye contact, and changes in body posture. When weight gain or loss, pregnancy, or injury visibly alters the client's or the therapist's body, there may be discussion of that fact, and of bodies, and a working through of meanings of that change, and possible related re-enactments. However, it is less common for most trauma therapists, even relational therapists, to comment on and inquire about the client's body, sexuality, or physical health. This omission is itself a dissociative process. We believe that understanding the process of dissociation is central to including successfully the client's (and the therapist's) body in trauma work, which is, in turn, essential to the client's recovery and well-being.

Theoretical Framework for Understanding Dissociation

Dissociation is a process in which an individual's awareness of various aspects of personal experience is not integrated. It is a separation of aspects of one's inner experience that allows someone not to know what seems to be obvious (Allen, 2001; Braun, 1988). Davies and Frawley (1994) described the process as "the last ditch effort of an overwhelmed ego to salvage some semblance of adequate mental functioning" (p. 65). Dissociation allows many children to survive psychologically by separating their minds from what is happening to their bodies. It is easy to see how this survival skill would naturally carry over into adulthood. Unfortunately, its adaptational value decreases significantly when the adult is disconnected from his or her physical well-being.

Our understanding of dissociation is based in constructivist self development theory (McCann & Pearlman, 1990; Pearlman & Saakvitne, 1995; Saakvitne et al., 2000), which describes aspects of the self that are affected by traumatic life experiences. One such aspect is the self-capacities or inner abilities to regulate internal psychological processes and experience. (See Pearlman, 1998, for an in-depth discussion of the role, development, and repair of self-capacities.) These capacities include the ability to regulate affect, maintain a sense of positive self-worth, and maintain an inner sense of connection to benign others; they are developed in the earliest relationships with central caregivers or attachment figures. When those important others are not attuned to the child, are physically or emotionally absent, or are abusive, the child's self-capacities are not adequately developed.

Underdeveloped self-capacities are a hallmark of complex trauma. It is likely that underdeveloped self-capacities have a central role in the affect dysregulation, dissociation, relationship difficulties, and somatization that are part of the complex-trauma adaptation. Thus, a central aspect of therapy for survivors of early, severe, or cumulative trauma is the development of self-capacities. This development is a long, slow process that can occur in a relationship in which re-enactments can occur and be identified, named, acknowledged, and processed. The result of such a process is a different outcome, one that has the potential to heal attachment injuries (*attachment trauma*; Allen, 2001), which ultimately is a way to prevent crises such as self-injury, suicidality, and revictimization. This approach to therapy is at the heart of relational trauma treatment (Pearlman & Courtois, in press; Pearlman, 1998; Saakvitne et al., 2000).

In adulthood, individuals with inadequately developed self-capacities struggle to tolerate or modulate their feelings. A familiar solution to this struggle for many survivors is dissociation, a response to potential or experienced danger that short-circuits feelings, whether the source is internal or external. Pearlman and Saakvitne (1995) explained the central importance of understanding dissociation both as an intrapsychic defense and, in psychotherapy, as an interpersonal process:

> Phenomenologically, it is the separation of mental systems that would ordinarily be integrated. It represents the severing of connections among mental contents and categories that would otherwise elaborate and augment one another. Theoretically, it provides the therapist an invaluable framework for understanding a range of intrapsychic and interpersonal occurrences in psychotherapy with trauma survivors. (p. 120)

Pearlman and Saakvitne (1995) continued by defining the intrapsychic functions of dissociation as follows: (a) to separate oneself from intolerable affects, reflecting the need not to feel; (b) to separate oneself from traumatic memories and knowledge, reflecting the need not to know; (c) to separate from unacceptable aspects of oneself, reflecting the need not to be oneself; and (d) to separate from the interpersonal relationship, reflecting the need to manage the threat that connection poses. (See Pearlman & Saakvitne, 1995, for an in-depth conceptualization and discussion of dissociation and countertransference responses.) Jane likely had underdeveloped self-capacities, and she seemed to have replaced her limited affect tolerance with dissociation for many years. As she encountered in the therapy new possibilities for relating and then for experiencing herself differently, her dissociation was no longer the first line of defense against previously intolerable thoughts and feelings.

Understanding dissociative processes and their functions is essential to bringing the client's physical experience to her or his awareness within the therapy relationship. When the therapist has a broader perspective on the client's physical experience—beyond psychological experiences of anxiety and stress, for example—she is in a position to invite the client to notice, take interest in, and name that physical experience. Although somatic concerns often do not have a physical etiology that can be treated medically, such an approach can lead to the possibility of obtaining medical care for the many physical illnesses that can be treated effectively. Jane's therapist might have brought a discussion of the dissociative processes and Jane's physical experience into the therapy as follows:

> Over the last several months, we've worked together to find ways to help you separate the past from the present during flashbacks. I have such admiration for your efforts to find language and name your experiences—like when you've talked about not being able to feel your feet. Sometimes when we're not working on past memories, I've noticed that you rub your ankles and seem to be in pain when you walk. Do your feet hurt?

Many trauma therapists have noted that dissociation is "contagious"; when the client is unaware of something, it is often difficult for the therapist to bring it to mind or keep it in her or his own awareness (Davies & Frawley, 1994; Pearlman & Saakvitne, 1995; Saakvitne et al., 2000). Therapists may be more comfortable in the moment not knowing about the horrible things that were done to the small bodies of helpless children. The not-knowing is one way some therapists automatically and naturally attempt to protect themselves from vicarious traumatization (McCann & Pearlman, 1990), although, like peritraumatic dissociation for victims, it seems likely to lead to more negative long-term consequences than would remaining present and connected (Forrester, 2001).

CHILDHOOD MALTREATMENT AND PHYSICAL HEALTH RESEARCH

A review of the relevant literature will provide some background for our approach to working with survivors on their physical health issues. Many individuals who endure early, severe abuse or neglect, or cumulative experiences of traumatic loss, abandonment, or exposure to violence, develop a range of adaptations that are described by the term *complex trauma* or *complex posttraumatic stress disorder* (Herman, 1992; Pelcovitz, van der Kolk, Roth, Mandel, Kaplan, & Resick, 1997). Recent developments in research and theory related to complex trauma have greatly advanced an understanding of its elements. These include revictimization (e.g., Cloitre, 1998; Nishith, Mechanic, & Resick, 2000; Roodman & Clum, 2001; Widom, 1999), affect dysregulation or hyperresponsiveness (Allen, 2001; Kendall-Tackett, 2000), relationship difficulties (Pearlman & Courtois, in press), identity and meaning (Harvey, 1996; Lantz, 1996), dissociation (Putnam, 1997; Waller et al., 2000), and somatization (Neumann, Houskamp, Pollock, & Briere, 1996; Nijenhuis, 2000).

Researchers and clinicians have conceptualized the physical health problems that accompany complex trauma in a variety of ways. The inclusion of somatization within the complex trauma rubric is one frame. Somatization can be conceptualized as the representation of psychological experiences through bodily experience, that is, physical illnesses or aches and pains whose origins are psychological. Nijenhuis and his colleagues (Nijenhuis, 2000) have expanded an understanding of somatization in trauma survivors, returning to Jane's original conceptualization of somatization as a form of dissociation. (See Laria & Lewis-Fernandez, 2001, for a review of the history of the relation between dissociation and somatization.) This conceptualization offers clinicians and clients a better understanding and opens new possibilities for addressing the experience and process of somatization. Somatization, however, is only one physical manifestation of childhood maltreatment.

There has also been excellent work in the past decade concerning the psychobiological effects of traumatic life experiences, contributions that have changed the way mental health professionals think about trauma (e.g., Shalev, Bleich, & Ursano, 1990; Schnurr et al., 2000; Yehuda & McFarlane, 1997; van der Kolk, 1994). In his seminal article, "The Body Keeps the Score" (1994), van der Kolk provided a significant frame for an understanding of stress-induced analgesia, noting that "the dissociative reactions in people in response to trauma may be analogous to the complex behaviors that occur in animals after prolonged exposure to severe uncontrollable stress" (p. 227). Originally, in research with severely stressed animals, and then in people with PTSD, researchers found that, when faced with inescapable stressors, the body activates the secretion of endogenous opioids, resulting in stress-induced analgesia. This research found that as much as 20 years after the original stressor, people with PTSD developed opioid-mediated analgesia in response to a stimulus resembling the traumatic stressor, which correlated with a secretion of endogenous opioids equivalent to 8 mg of morphine (Pitman, van der Kolk, Orr, & Greenberg, 1990; van der Kolk, Greenberg, Orr, & Pitman, 1989).

In our work with trauma survivors, this concept significantly broadens our understanding of and response to two central and familiar adaptations. First, as noted by van der Kolk (1994) and others, the dissociative process of self-harm may, for some survivors, serve as a conditioned stimulus for the release of endogenous opioids and the resulting feeling of calm. The understanding by client and therapist of the physiologically addictive nature of tissue self-injury can reduce the shame and humiliation that often accompany self-injury and provide richer opportunities to respectfully name, normalize, and address the self-harming behavior (Davies & Frawley, 1994; Miller, 1994). Second, changes in pain perception can be affected by this "natural" analgesia. It seems reasonable to consider this finding as a way of understanding the increased tolerance to pain we witness in many clients who use dissociation as a primary adaptation, an observation borne out by recent research (Nijenhuis, Spinhoven, Vanderlinden, van Dyck, & van der Hart, 1998). "Nature provides protection against pain by means of [stress-induced analgesia]" (van der Kolk, 1994, p. 227). This initial protection against feeling pain from abuse-related injuries, if sustained through the dissociative process, may result in years of unrecognized or minimized medical problems. A study of altered pain perception in women with gastrointestinal disorders and a history of abuse noted, "Given that victims of abuse tend to blame themselves for the occurrence of the abusive acts, it is not surprising that abused patients also tend to take responsibility for their pain" (Scarinci, McDonald-Haile, Bradley, & Richter, 1994, p. 116).

The medical literature, coming from another perspective, has thoroughly documented the long-term adverse health effects of child maltreatment (e.g., Felitti et al., 1998; McCauley et al., 1997). Physical effects of abuse can include scars, limb and spine deformities due to fractures, and sensory impairment. These effects are often exacerbated by the lack of adequate medical attention to abuse-related injuries (Loewenstein & Goodwin, 1999; Rosenberg & Krugman, 1991). Weiner (1992) used the term *ill health* to capture the many complaints that survivors bring to physicians without finding adequate explanations. Allen (2001) explored these findings and conceptualizations as they apply to our work with survivor clients. He recommended conceptualizing PTSD as a chronic physical illness, using diabetes as a paradigm and providing education about self-care as a foundation for these psychotherapies. Additional recent contributions to an understanding of trauma and the body include *Waking the Tiger* (Levine, 1997), *Splintered Reflections* (Goodwin & Attias, 1999), and *The Body Remembers* (Rothschild, 2000).

Friedman and Schnurr (1995) offered another important perspective on the relation between trauma and physical health. They noted that in response to PTSD symptoms, many survivors engage in behaviors that further endanger their health, such as cigarette smoking or substance overuse, to manage anxiety. In a major study in a large health maintenance organization, Felitti et al. (1998) found that people with four or more adverse childhood experiences, compared to those with none, had a four- to twelvefold increased risk for drug abuse and alcoholism and a two- to fourfold increase in risk for smoking, sexually transmitted diseases, and more sexual partners.

All of this research points in one direction: Childhood abuse and neglect create physical devastation. This observation converges with our deepening clinical understanding that dissociation may be one of the primary ways survivors tolerate that impact on their bodies. As psychotherapists attempting to help survivor clients piece together their experiences, we attend exquisitely to the nuances of past and present. We need to use our relational skills and theoretical base to help clients also weave together the various aspects of their present experience, including mind, body, and spirit.

CONCLUSION

Jane and her therapist resumed therapy sessions about three weeks after her heart procedure, as soon as Jane felt physically able. The first session very poignantly demonstrated the power of a relational trauma therapy to begin to shift a trauma survivor's options to dissociative processes:

Jane: Well, I really messed up this time.

Therapist: Can you help me understand how you feel you messed up, Jane?

Jane: The doctor said the problem with my heart has been around for awhile and that I have to reduce my stress. He also said there are other problems with my body. I thought I was doing a good job of taking care of things.

Therapist: Taking care of everything and keeping things separate at the same time was the way you learned to survive and protect yourself through absolutely horrible situations and abuse. You learned to dissociate to make your way through an impossible dilemma.

Jane: I just keep thinking about how stupid I was not to put it together.

Therapist: I know that feeling stupid and responsible is very familiar and has kept away other feelings that haven't seemed safe. I've been so reminded over these past three weeks of the times in here that you've told me that your heart hurt and how we both connected to your feelings of loss but not the signs that there might also be a physical problem.

Jane: (She is beginning to cry and lowering her head.) So I really wasn't alone in not figuring it out? You didn't know either?

Therapist: No, Jane, you weren't alone. I wish I had connected the possibility of a physical problem, just like I wish I had been able to stop what happened to you as a child. I'm sorry you have been alone with so many things, and I hope you and I can continue to work together and learn from each other to help you heal.

Our hope in writing this chapter is for both medical and psychological trauma researchers to include a focus on dissociation and physical health in their work with complex trauma survivor clients. Although the concept of somatic dissociation is receiving excellent renewed attention in the literature, it is essential that it not obscure one's view of the direct physical health consequences of physical abuse and neglect. Trauma survivor clients could benefit greatly—in terms of reduced morbidity, shame, and fear—from increased dialogue between mental health and physical health care providers.

We encourage psychotherapists to become aware of the importance of including conversation about the client's body and physical health in psychotherapies with childhood trauma survivor clients. A solid grounding in theory, research, and practice—including talking with clients and supervisors about these issues—will help members of the field to develop a language and comfort with exploring trauma and physical health. Therapists may learn to attend differently to what clients are saying about their bodies and health. They may be more effective in providing psychoeducational information to their clients, as well as in learning from them, about the possible physical effects of childhood neglect and abuse.

REFERENCES

Allen, J. G. (2001). *Traumatic relationships and serious mental disorders*. West Sussex, England: Wiley.

Braun, B. G. (1988). The BASK model of dissociation. *Dissociation, 11*, 4–23.

Briere, J., & Gil, E. (1998). Self-mutilation in clinical and general population samples: Prevalence, correlates, and functions. *American Journal of Orthopsychiatry, 68*, 609–620.

Cloitre, M. (1998). Sexual revictimization: Risk factors and prevention. In V. M. Follette, J. I. Ruzek, & F. R. Abueg (Eds.), *Cognitive–behavioral therapies for trauma* (pp. 278–304). New York: Guilford Press.

Connors, R. E. (2000). *Self-injury: Psychotherapy with people who engage in self-inflicted violence*. Northvale, NJ: Jason Aronson.

Davies, J. M., & Frawley, M. G. (1994). *Treating the adult survivor of childhood sexual abuse: A psychoanalytic perspective*. New York: Basic Books.

Felitti, V. J., Anda, R. F., Nordenberg, D., Williamson, D. F., Spitz, A. M., Edwards, V., et al. (1998). Relationship of childhood abuse and household dysfunction to many of the leading causes of death in adults: The Adverse Childhood Experiences (ACE) study. *American Journal of Preventive Medicine, 14*, 245–258.

Forrester, C. A. (2001, December). *Body awareness, countertransference, and vicarious traumatization*. Poster presented at the 17th annual meeting of the International Society for Traumatic Stress Studies, New Orleans, LA.

Friedman, M. J., & Schnurr, P. P. (1995). The relationship between trauma, posttraumatic stress disorder, and physical health. In M. J. Friedman, D. S. Charney, & A. Y. Deutch (Eds.), *Neurobiological and clinical consequences of stress: From normal adaptation to post-traumatic stress disorder* (pp. 507–524). Philadelphia: Lippincott-Raven.

Goodwin, J. M., & Attias, R. (1999). *Splintered reflections: Images of the body in trauma.* New York: Basic Books.

Harvey, M. (1996). An ecological view of psychological trauma and trauma recovery. *Journal of Traumatic Stress, 9,* 3–23.

Herman, J. L. (1992). Complex PTSD: A syndrome in survivors of prolonged and repeated trauma. *Journal of Traumatic Stress, 5,* 377–391.

Jordan, J. V., Kaplan, A. G., Miller, J. B., Stiver, I. P., & Surrey, J. L. (1991). *Women's growth in connection: Writings from the Stone Center.* Wellesley, MA: Stone Center Working Paper Series.

Kendall-Tackett, K. A. (2000). Physiological correlates of childhood abuse: Chronic hyperarousal in PTSD, depression, and irritable bowel syndrome. *Child Abuse and Neglect, 24,* 799–810.

Lantz, J. (1996). Logotherapy as trauma therapy. *Crisis Intervention and Time-Limited Treatment, 2,* 243–253.

Laria, A. J., & Lewis-Fernandez, R. (2001). The professional fragmentation of experience in the study of dissociation, somatization, and culture. *Journal of Trauma and Dissociation, 2,* 17–47.

Levine, P. A. (1997). *Waking the tiger: Healing trauma.* Berkeley, CA: North Atlantic.

Loewenstein, R. J., & Goodwin, J. M. (1999). Assessment and management of somatoform symptoms in traumatized patients: Conceptual overview and pragmatic guide. In J. M. Goodwin & R. Attias (Eds.), *Splintered reflections: Images of the body in trauma* (pp. 67–88). New York: Basic Books.

McCann, I. L., & Pearlman, L. A. (1990). *Psychological trauma and the adult survivor: Theory, therapy, and transformation.* New York: Brunner/Mazel.

McCauley, J., Kern, E. E., Kolodner, K., Dill, L., Schroeder, A. F., DeChant, H. K., et al. (1997). Clinical characteristics of women with a history of childhood abuse. *Journal of the American Medical Association, 277,* 1362–1368.

Miller, D. (1994). *Women who hurt themselves: A book of hope and understanding.* New York: Basic Books.

Neumann, D. A., Houskamp, B. M., Pollock, V. E., & Briere, J. (1996). The long-term sequelae of childhood sexual abuse in women: A meta-analytic review. *Child Maltreatment, 1,* 6–16.

Nicholls, S. S., Deiter, P. J., & Pearlman, L. A. (2000). *Self-harming behaviors and reasons for self-harm.* Unpublished manuscript.

Nijenhuis, E. R. S. (2000). Somatoform dissociation: Major symptoms of dissociative disorders. *Journal of Trauma and Dissociation, 1,* 7–32.

Nijenhuis, E. R. S., Spinhoven, P., Vanderlinden, J., van Dyck, R., & van der Hart., O. (1998). Somatoform dissociative symptoms as related to animal defensive reactions to predatory imminence and injury. *Journal of Abnormal Psychology, 107,* 63–73.

Nijenhuis, E. R. S., Vanderlinden, J., & Spinhoven, P. (1998). Animal defensive reactions as a model for trauma-induced dissociative reactions. *Journal of Traumatic Stress, 11,* 243–260.

Nishith, P., Mechanic, M. B., & Resick, P. A. (2000). Prior interpersonal trauma: The contribution to current PTSD symptoms in female rape victims. *Journal of Abnormal Psychology, 109,* 20–25.

Pearlman, L. A. (1998). Trauma and the self: A theoretical and clinical perspective. *Journal of Emotional Abuse, 1,* 7–25.

Pearlman, L. A., & Courtois, C. A. (in press). Clinical applications of the attachment framework: Relational treatment of complex trauma. *Journal of Traumatic Stress.*

Pearlman, L. A., & Saakvitne, K. W. (1995). *Trauma and the therapist: Countertransference and vicarious traumatization in psychotherapy with incest survivors.* New York: Norton.

Pelcovitz, D., van der Kolk, B. A., Roth, S. H., Mandel, F. S., Kaplan, S. J., & Resick, P. A. (1997). Development of a criteria set and a structured interview for disorders of extreme stress (SIDES). *Journal of Traumatic Stress, 10,* 3–16.

Pitman, R. K., van der Kolk, B. A., Orr, S. P., & Greenberg, M. S. (1990). Naloxone-reversible stress-induced analgesia in posttraumatic stress disorder. *Archives of General Psychiatry, 47,* 541–547.

Putnam, F. W. (1997). *Dissociation in children and adolescents: A developmental perspective.* New York: Guilford Press.

Roodman, A. A., & Clum, G. A. (2001). Revictimization rates and method variance: A meta-analysis. *Clinical Psychology Review, 21,* 183–204.

Rosenberg, D. A., & Krugman, R. D. (1991). Epidemiology and outcome of child abuse. *Annual Review of Medicine, 42,* 217–224.

Rothschild, B. (2000). *The body remembers: The psychophysiology of trauma and trauma treatment.* New York: Norton.

Saakvitne, K. W., Gamble, S. G., Pearlman, L. A., & Lev, B. T. (2000). *Risking connection: A training curriculum for working with survivors of childhood abuse.* Lutherville, MD: Sidran Foundation.

Santa Mina, E. E., & Gallop, R. M. (1998). Childhood sexual and physical abuse and adult self-harm and suicidal behaviour: A literature review. *Canadian Journal of Psychiatry, 43,* 793–800.

Scarinci, I. C., McDonald-Haile, J., Bradley, L. A., & Richter, J. E. (1994). Altered pain perception and psychosocial features among women with gastrointestinal disorders and history of abuse: A preliminary model. *American Journal of Medicine, 97,* 108–118.

Schnurr, P. P., Spiro, A. III, & Paris, A. H. (2000). Physician-diagnosed medical disorders in relation to PTSD symptoms in older male military veterans. *Health Psychology, 19,* 91–97.

Shalev, A., Bleich, A., & Ursano, R. J. (1990). Posttraumatic stress disorder: Somatic comorbidity and effort tolerance. *Psychosomatics, 31,* 197–203.

van der Kolk, B. (1994). The body keeps the score: Memory and the evolving psychobiology of posttraumatic stress. *Harvard Review of Psychiatry, 1*, 253–265.

van der Kolk, B. A., Greenberg, M. S., Orr, S. P., & Pitman, R. K. (1989). Endogenous opioids and stress induced analgesia in posttraumatic stress disorder. *Psychopharmacology Bulletin, 25*, 108–112.

Waller, G., Hamilton, K., Elliott, P., Lewwendon, J., Stopa, L., Waters, A., et al. (2000). Somatoform dissociation, psychological dissociation, and specific forms of trauma. *Journal of Trauma and Dissociation, 1*, 81–98.

Weiner, H. (1992). *Perturbing the organism: The biology of stressful experience*. Chicago: University of Chicago Press.

Widom, C. S. (1999). Posttraumatic stress disorder in abused and neglected children grown up. *American Journal of Psychiatry, 156*, 1223–1229.

Yehuda, R., & McFarlane, A. C. (Eds.). (1997). *Psychobiology of posttraumatic stress disorder*. New York: New York Academy of Sciences.

Zlotnick, C., Shea, M. T., Pearlstein, T., Simpson, E., Costello, E., & Begin, A. (1996). The relationship between dissociative symptoms, alexithymia, impulsivity, sexual abuse, and self-mutilation. *Comprehensive Psychiatry, 37*, 12–16.

13

BATTERED WOMEN AND TRAUMATIC BRAIN INJURY

HELENE JACKSON, ELIZABETH PHILIP, RONALD L. NUTTALL,
AND LEONARD DILLER

The inability of substantial numbers of battered women to terminate or extricate themselves from violent relationships is of grave concern to clinical practitioners. Despite professional intervention, many victims of domestic violence return to the batterer and to repetitive battering, demonstrating that, for these women, traditional psychosocial interventions are ineffective. In a sample of 53 battered women, 92% reported having received blows to the head in the course of their battering; 40% reported loss of consciousness. Correlations between frequency of being hit in the head and severity of cognitive symptoms were significant, strongly suggesting that battered women should be routinely screened for traumatic brain injury and postconcussive syndrome. Development of treatment strategies to address the potentially damaging sequelae of head trauma in this population is essential.

Reprinted from "Traumatic Brain Injury: A Hidden Consequence for Batterd Women," by H. Jackson, E. Philip, R. L. Nuttall, and L. Diller, 2002, *Professional Psychology: Research and Practice*, 33, pp. 39–45. Copyright 2002 by the American Psychological Association. Reprinted with permission.

Clinicians are frequently unaware of the incidence of head injury sustained by battered women in the course of their battering. Consequently, the damaging sequelae of such trauma are often misdiagnosed (National Institutes of Health [NIH], 1999). According to a 1986 national survey of family violence (Straus & Gelles, 1986), 6% of American women have been severely assaulted by their male partners in any given year. Typical injuries range from being punched, kicked, choked, beaten, and threatened or assaulted with a knife or gun (Straus, 1990). Despite professional intervention, significant numbers of battered women return to the batterer and to repetitive battering (Walker, 1991), often leading to serious injury or death (Wilt, Illman, & Field, 1997). Yet our understanding of how best to treat victims of domestic violence remains incomplete.

In this chapter, we show that significant numbers of battered women may suffer from the sequelae of head injury. We recommend that battered women be routinely screened for traumatic brain injury (TBI) and postconcussive syndrome (PCS) and, where appropriate, referred for neuropsychological testing. Identification of women whose behavior may be an indication of neurological rather than, or in addition to, psychological, sociological, and environmental factors has major implications for the treatment of battered women.

In 1991, Walker observed that battered women frequently demonstrate "neurological signs that appear to have been caused by repeated head injuries" (p. 25). Although there has recently been interest in the relationship between TBI and the assaultive behavior of batterers (Rosenbaum et al., 1994), Walker's observations and the link between TBI and symptoms associated with battered women have not been systematically explored until now.

Here we examine the prevalence of mild traumatic brain injury (MTBI), sometimes referred to as *minor head injury, concussion,* or *posttraumatic syndrome* (T. Kay, 1992). We discuss the relationship between MTBI and symptoms commonly observed in battered women who have sustained repetitive assaults to the head and face (Ochs, Neuenschwander, & Dodson, 1996), and we distinguish between MTBI, the injury that results from blows to the head, and PCS, a complex set of physical, cognitive, behavioral, and affective complaints observed in some MTBI patients (American Psychiatric Association [APA], 1994). TBI has been defined as "a subset of minor head injury in which damage to the head includes damage to the brain" that can result in symptoms that may or may not be transient (R. Kay, Newman, Cavallo, Ezrachi, & Resnick, 1992, p. 372). Suggested criteria for PCS are loss of consciousness (immediate to the injury) lasting for more than 5 min, posttraumatic amnesia for more than 12 hr postinjury, evidence of cognitive deficits in concentration, shifting focus of attention, and difficulty performing simultaneous cognitive tasks beginning within 6 months of injury (APA,

1994). However, recent research conducted by Lovell, Iverson, Collins, McKeag, and Maroon (1999) showed no relationship between traumatic loss of consciousness and neuropsychological functioning, suggesting that loss of consciousness may not be a reliable criterion on which to base a diagnosis of PCS. Lovell et al. found that patients who had sustained traumatic loss of consciousness were no more likely to perform poorly on neuropsychological tests shown to be sensitive to MTBI than were patients who had no or uncertain loss of consciousness (Lovell et al., 1999).

Symptoms of PCS may include any three or more of the following that persist for at least 3 months postinjury: easy fatigue, sleep disorder, headaches, dizziness, irritability or aggression, anxiety, depression or affective lability, lack of spontaneity, and changes in social or sexual behavior (APA, 1994). Among the factors affecting the likelihood of developing prolonged PCS are repeated concussions, such as those sustained by boxers, football, and soccer players (NIH, 1999); family and social stress; and unrealistic expectations that the individual prematurely return to his or her premorbid level of functioning (Gronwall, 1989). Because a history of MTBI is not usually documented in medical records, many such injuries go unrecognized, and prevalence is underestimated (NIH, 1999).

Among the syndromes and psychiatric disorders associated with battered women, the most frequent are battered woman syndrome (Pelcovitz et al., 1997; Walker, 1977-1978; 1994), depression (Gelles & Straus, 1990), and posttraumatic stress syndrome (PTSD; Sutherland, Bybee, & Sullivan, 1998). Although individuals with MTBI may exhibit symptoms consistent with PTSD, studies have shown that the full criteria required for a diagnosis of PTSD are rarely met (R. Kay et al., 1992). For battered women who are seen in emergency rooms, the majority of injuries are located on the head and face (Ochs et al., 1996), suggesting a possible relationship between MTBI and symptoms observed in battered women. Cognitive and memory distortions, amnesia and dissociation (Slagle, 1990), depression, irritability, isolation, and avoidance (Sutherland et al., 1998), often attributed to PTSD, are consistent with a diagnosis of PCS.

Like MTBI patients, many battered women demonstrate an inability to pay attention (Ferrant, 1992). They may frequently have difficulty with any combination of the following: concentration, feeling confused, poor judgment (Sato & Heiby, 1992), problem solving (Claerhout, Elder, & Janes, 1982), and decision making (Browne, 1993). Like MTBI patients, severely battered women are likely to complain of frequent headaches and experience serious memory problems (Gelles & Straus, 1990). They may be depressed and have pervasive feelings of being overwhelmed (Stark & Flitcraft, 1996).

Until the 1960s, it was believed that symptoms associated with MTBI were transitory and reversible; those who continued to complain were labeled neurotic or malingerers. However, recent research has shown that for some, the "time frame common to the majority" is not germane (Dikman, Temkin, & Armsden, 1989, p. 237). Mild traumatic brain injury can produce "long-term damage . . . which may not be apparent in normal circumstances, but which is evident when the system is stressed" (Gronwall, 1989, p. 161). Accordingly, the sequelae of MTBI may "endure in original or altered forms across the lifespan, with new problems likely to occur as a result of new challenges and the aging process" (NIH, 1999, p. 976). Studies of MTBI have shown that about 10% of those injured continue to manifest PCS one year postinjury and that these symptoms, once established, "do not spontaneously remit" (R. Kay et al., 1992, p. 373).

According to the NIH (1999) Consensus Panel, long-term cognitive consequences of MTBI may include memory impairment; attention and concentration limitations; language deficits; and difficulties in problem solving, abstract thinking, insight, judgment, planning, information processing, and organization. Behavioral difficulties may include verbal and physical aggression, lack of insight, sexual dysfunction, depression, and anxiety. Social sequelae may include increased risk of suicide, divorce, chronic unemployment, financial stress, and substance abuse. Early identification of MTBI can minimize the development of these complications (Kelly, 1975) and may be cost-effective in decreasing time lost from school or work (Lawler & Terregino, 1996). Currently, battered women are not routinely screened for MTBI, and current treatment interventions do not reflect this etiology.

BATTERED WOMEN AND THE MTBI SURVEY

The aim of this pilot study was to investigate, in a sample of battered women, the prevalence of MTBI (independent variable) and the frequency and severity of symptoms consistent with PCS (dependent variables). Sixty-eight women attending support groups at three battered women's shelters and four community outreach programs were asked by staff members, over a 2-week period in January 1997 if they were interested in participating in a study about domestic violence. Women were assured of complete anonymity and told that their decision would not affect their or their children's access to, or quality of, services. All data were obtained by self-report.

Fifty-three women (77.9% of those eligible; 36 living in three shelters, 17 attending four community outreach programs) consented to participate by returning completed, anonymous questionnaires in sealed envelopes. Ages of the participants ranged from 18 to 48 years, with a mean age of 30 years ($SD = 7$). About a third (36%) had less than a high school degree; 43% were high school graduates. Although 21% had some college education, none had graduated. Most (86%) were unemployed; almost half (45%) were married; 26% were single, never married; 21% were separated or divorced; and 8% were living with a partner. Most (60%) were African American; 28% were Hispanic; 6% Caucasian; 4% Native American; and 2% Asian. Forty-three percent were Catholic; 34% Protestant; 4% Muslim; and 2% Jewish; 17% endorsed no religion.

The choice of an instrument to screen for brain injury in a population of battered women presents major challenges. Because the majority of respondents in this study were residents of a battered women's shelter, measures such as the Glasgow Coma Scale (Teasdale & Jennet, 1974), which must be administered immediately after the trauma, could not be used. Furthermore, unlike other brain-injured populations seen in emergency departments, the majority of whom are men injured in automobile accidents (Silver, Hales, & Yudofsky, 1994), many battered women are likely to have suffered repetitive, rather than single-event, head trauma (Walker, 1991). They may not recognize their symptoms to be a result of their injuries and consequently are unlikely to seek treatment for head trauma immediate to an assault.

To screen for the possibility of head injury, we used the HELPS questionnaire. A brief, preliminary screening tool developed by a team of head trauma specialists (Picard, Scarisbrick, & Paluck, 1999), the HELPS questionnaire is designed for use by professionals not trained in neurology to identify patients in need of in-depth neuropsychological assessment. It is short, easy to use, and sensitive to the target areas. Although its psychometric properties are not known, the HELPS inclusion criteria are consistent with generally established medical parameters identified in the brain injury literature—for example, loss of consciousness and PCS (Silver, Yudofsky, & Hales, 1994). On the basis of evidence that noncontact intracranial brain movement, such as whiplash or severe shaking, can cause diffuse brain injuries that may result in cognitive and functional deficits (NIH, 1999), we added questions about severe shaking to the questionnaire.

We limited the criteria for MTBI to either or both (a) a blow to the head with loss of consciousness or (b) alterations in consciousness (confusion, posttraumatic amnesia, dizziness, nausea) following the injury (T. Kay et al., 1993). Our criteria for PCS subsequent to MTBI included any 3 or more of 13 cognitive symptoms commonly associated with MTBI and included in the HELPS questionnaire (see Table 13.1).

To measure the severity of symptoms, we developed a Total Symptom Severity Index (TSSI) by averaging scores across all 13 symptoms for each of the three time frames for answers to the question, "Do you have [this symptom]?" Possible response categories were coded as 0 (no, I don't have this problem), 1 (yes, I have had this problem in the last 5 years), 2 (yes, I have had this problem in the past year), or 3 (yes, I have this problem currently). Thus, the lowest possible score per time frame (0.0) corresponds to having no symptoms; the highest (3.0) corresponds to having all 13 symptoms.

TABLE 13.1
Time Distribution of Postconcussive Symptoms of 53 Battered Women

Symptom	None	In past 5 years[a]	In past year[b]	Current[c]
Easily distracted	19	2	13	66
Trouble concentrating	23	2	11	64
Trouble remembering[d]	28	0	9	62
Trouble paying attention to more than one thing	25	0	13	62
Trouble in distracting environment	26	0	17	57
Forgetting appointments[a]	23	0	21	57
Trouble doing more than one thing at a time	34	0	13	53
Headaches	17	11	19	53
Difficulty finding the right words	34	2	17	47
Losing things	40	2	13	45
Work became harder[e]	40	2	19	40
Dizziness	36	7	38	19
Trouble following directions	74	0	13	13

Note. Numbers are percentages. [a] Exclusive of past year and current categories. [b] Exclusive of current category. [c] Exclusive of past year category. [d] Differences in percentages between Tables 13.1 and 13.2 are a result of missing data. [e] Adds to more than 100% as a result of rounding numbers.

Symptom severity scores for the third category (*yes, I have this problem currently*) ranged from 0.00 to 2.85, with a mean of 1.83 (*SD* = 0.85). The Cronbach alpha coefficient for the 13 symptoms of the TSSI was .89, indicating high reliability.

To measure the current frequency of each of the 13 symptoms, we also developed a Total Symptom Frequency Index (TSFI). Respondents were asked, "Do you have [this symptom]?" If no, the symptom was coded as 0. If yes, respondents were asked, "How often does this happen?" Possible response categories were coded as 5 (*more than once a day*), 4 (*at least once a day*), 3 (*at least once a week*), 2 (*at least once a month*), and 1 (*less than once a month*). The Cronbach alpha coefficient for the TSFI of the current 13 symptoms was .92, indicating very high reliability. Pearson product–moment correlations were calculated to measure the relationships among the TSFI and having been hit in the head or shaken, duration of loss of consciousness, and the dependent variable (TSSI).

Forty-nine (92%) of the 53 women reported a history of having been hit in the head or face during partner violence. Of the total sample, 91% reported having been hit in the head in the "past year" category, with a mode frequency of 2–5 times. In the "past 5 years" category (2–5 years inclusive), 88% reported having been hit in the head by their partners, also with a mode of 2–5 times. Of the total sample, 25% (*n* = 13) reported

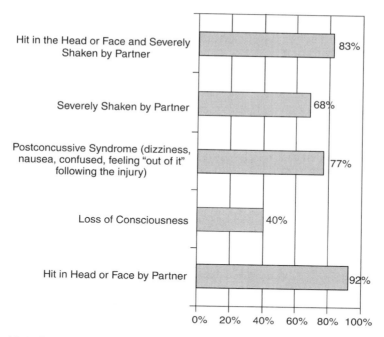

Figure 13.1. Battering history of 53 women.

having been hit in the head or face more than 20 times in the "past 5 years" category; 8% (*n* = 4) reported this high frequency in the "past year" category.

Forty percent (*n* = 21) of the women reported at least one instance when they were aware that they had lost consciousness as a result of having been hit in the head or face or severely shaken by a partner; 13% (*n* = 7) reported 2–4 such episodes. Duration of loss of consciousness ranged from "less than 1 min" to "30 min" (mode = 1–5 min). Seventy-seven percent of the total sample (*n* = 41) reported symptoms consistent with PCS following the assault—that is, dizziness, memory gaps, nausea, confusion, and feeling "out of it" (see Figure 13.1).

The majority of women reported frequent and acute cognitive difficulties, including current problems with being easily distracted; forgetting appointments; having headaches; and having trouble concentrating, paying attention, remembering things, and doing more than one thing at a time (see Table 13.1). In summary, roughly half of the women reported about half of the 13 symptoms one or more times a day. The frequencies with which women reported experiencing the 13 symptoms within the "past year" category ranged from 9% (trouble remembering) to 38% (dizziness; see Tables 13.1 and 13.2).

TABLE 13.2
Frequency Distribution of Current Symptoms of 53 Battered Women

Symptom	None	Less than 1/month	At least 1/month	At least 1/week	At least 1/day	More than 1/day
Easily distracted	17	2	2	11	33	35
Trouble concentrating	23	4	2	9	24	38
Trouble remembering things	30	0	8	6	24	32
Trouble paying attention to more than one thing	24	2	6	8	15	45
Trouble in distracting environment	26	4	7	17	15	30
Forgetting appointments	23	11	13	40	9	4
Trouble doing more than one thing at a time	34	4	2	11	15	34
Headaches	17	4	8	34	26	11
Difficulty finding the right words[a]	34	2	6	17	21	21
Losing things	40	0	11	36	11	2
Work became harder[b]	32	0	2	17	23	25
Dizziness	36	2	21	28	9	4
Trouble following directions[a]	74	4	13	4	6	0

Note. Numbers are percentages.
[a] Adds to more than 100% because of rounding numbers.   [b] Differences in percentages between Tables 13.1 and 13.2 are a result of missing data.

We found a statistically significant relationship between having lost consciousness and symptomatology, ψ^2 (1, $N = 53$) = 6.35, $r = .35$, $p = .02$. Of the 21 women who reported a loss of consciousness, 20 (95%) reported symptoms consistent with PCS. Of the 32 women who did not report a loss of consciousness, 21 (68%) reported such symptoms.

Frequency of severe shaking by a partner ranged from once to "more than 20 times." Two thirds of the women ($n = 36$) reported having been severely shaken by their partners. Sixty-six percent ($n = 35$) reported such episodes in the "past year" category; 64% ($n = 34$) reported severe shaking in the "past 5 years" category. For both time periods, more than 20% ($n = 26$) reported frequencies ranging from 6 to more than 20 incidents.

A history of having been severely shaken by a partner at any time within the 5 years was correlated with the TSSI at .30 ($p = .03$), as was the frequency of having been severely shaken in the "past year" category. The correlation between the frequency of having been severely shaken in the "past 5 years" category and the TSSI was .34 ($p = .02$). The correlation between loss of consciousness as a result of having been hit in the head or severely shaken and the TSSI was .29 ($p = .04$).

In general, and not surprisingly, the more that the women had been hit in the head or face by their partners, the greater were their TSSI scores ($r = .33$, $p = .02$), similar to a "dose–response" relationship. The correlation between the frequency of having been hit in the head or face by a partner in the "past year" category and the TSSI was .31 ($p = .03$). The correlation between the frequency of having been hit in the head or face by a partner in the "past 5 years" category and the TSSI was .29 ($p = .04$).

The TSFI was, of course, highly correlated with the TSSI, $r = .95$, $p < .01$. As expected, the correlations between the TSFI and the battering history variables were similar to those of the TSSI: TSFI and having been hit in the head or face, $r = .28$, $p < .05$; TSFI and number of times hit in the head during the past year, $r = .28$, $p < .05$; TSFI and number of times hit in the head during the past 5 years, $r = .34$, $p < .05$; TSFI and ever shaken by partner, $r = .23$ (ns); and TSFI and times shaken by partner, $r = .29$, $p < .05$. We found no significant differences between the different ethnic and racial groups in either symptom severity or frequency.

The small sample size, selection bias, overrepresentation of lower socio-economic status and of minorities, and the retrospective nature of the reports limit the generalizability of our findings to the general population of battered women. Therefore, the data reported here should be viewed with caution. Despite evidence of a strong correlation between self-reported symptomatology and neurobehavioral dysfunction (Bohnen, Jolles, & Twijnstra, 1992), reliance on self-report requires careful interpretation. In this sample, the nature of head trauma and postconcussive symptomatology makes the task of accurately assessing past symptoms and their strength particularly difficult.

Although research shows that some individuals who report symptoms subsequent to head injury may be malingering in order to benefit in a lawsuit (Dikman et al., 1989), such motivation is highly unlikely in this sample. First, there is no evidence that any of the 53 respondents were involved in lawsuits; second, even had they been, the anonymous nature of the data collection would make it impossible for it to be used to support such litigation.

The incidence of MTBI identified in this study and the symptoms consistent with PCS may differ from that found in the general population of battered women. On the one hand, those who seek refuge in shelters may manifest the most damaging sequelae of battering. On the other hand, women who are sufficiently organized to complete the tasks required to enter the shelter system may represent the women who are the most cognitively intact and the least brain injured.

Although statistically significant, the correlations between the TSSI and indices of severity of blows to the head are not high, indicating that premorbid factors, the natural evolution of the aftereffects of MTBI, or the time since the trauma, may be contributing to the total symptomatology. However, the family and social stress characteristically experienced by battered women, the repetitive blows to the head, and the frequency with which women in this study reported current symptoms suggest that, for some, the symptoms may be a reflection of prolonged PCS (Collins et al., 1999; Gronwall, 1989; NIH, 1999).

The acute and chronic symptoms reported here (see Tables 13.1 and 13.2) are like those observed in boxers and in soccer and football players who have experienced repeated head trauma and for whom, to prevent the potential for further damage, safety procedures have recently been implemented (Matser, Kessels, Lezak, Jordan, & Troost, 1999; Powell & Barber-Foss, 1999). Battered women, like these athletes, become more symptomatic the more that they are hit in the head. Furthermore, dose–response relationships are considered powerful indicators of causal relationships in nonexperimental studies (Kubzansky et al., 1997; Southern, Smith, & Palmer, 1990), providing evidence in this study for the link between battering and postconcussive symptoms.

This study should be replicated with a more diverse sample of battered women from a variety of settings and expanded to include extensive neurological testing and follow-up to (a) examine, longitudinally, the association between MTBI and symptoms commonly observed in battered women and their evolution; (b) compare behaviors in a group of battered women with MTBI to a group of nonbattered women with MTBI and to a group of battered women who have sustained physical injuries other than MTBI; and (c) measure the relationships among PTSD, depression, and MTBI.

The frequency and severity of symptoms reported here would make it difficult to think through or cope with the complex, often formidable organizational tasks required for battered women to stop the violence, disengage from violent partners, and establish independent lives (Eby, Campbell, Sullivan, & Davidson, 1995). Thus, despite intervention, women who have sustained MTBI may be even less able than others to extricate themselves from abusive relationships.

PRACTICAL IMPLICATIONS

Recognition of MTBI as a hidden consequence of battering requires a multidisciplinary approach to prevent, whenever possible, the potentially dire consequences of future assaults (Matser et al., 1999). Those who see domestic violence victims should become familiar with the indicators of MTBI and PCS and knowledgeable about the neurophysiological risk factors associated with domestic violence and its dynamics. Women identified as battered should be screened routinely for traumatic brain injury, including direct questioning about the onset, frequency, and duration of blows to the head and face, severe shaking, loss of consciousness, and the presence of symptoms consistent with PCS.

Because this is a new area of investigation, there are no empirically derived guidelines to help the practitioner not trained in neurology determine whether a patient's screening indicates the probability of PCS. However, on the basis of the MTBI literature (T. Kay et al., 1993) and the authors' (E. Philip and L. Diller) clinical observations, we consider women to be at risk when they have a history of head injury and are currently experiencing three or more symptoms, at least once a day, that interfere with their daily functioning. Given the dose–response effect discussed earlier and the findings in the MTBI literature, practitioners should particularly attend to a history of repetitive assaults to the head and face and reports of headaches or dizziness. When screening is positive, referral for extensive neuropsychological testing to measure the patient's attention, concentration, memory, verbal capacity, and executive functioning is indicated (NIH, 1999). To minimize the potential for PCS, practitioners should caution patients to protect themselves against the likelihood of another head injury (Gronwall, 1989).

When neurological testing is positive, interventions must be designed to address the patient's cognitive, affective, and social impairments. They should be "individually tailored, structured, systematic [and] goal directed" (NIH, 1999, p. 979). Although there have been no systematic efforts to examine the effectiveness of psychotherapy in the MTBI population, NIH endorses its inclusion as an essential component of treatment.

Accordingly, we recommend some combination of psychosocial and rehabilitation treatment designed to do the following: address safety issues, enhance patients' self-esteem, furnish emotional support, provide education about head injury and its effects, reduce isolation, strengthen cognitive capacities to process and interpret information, improve ability to cope with everyday aspects of family and community life, provide information about available resources, and, when necessary, assist patients in "navigating" the health and rehabilitation systems (Diller, 1992; NIH, 1999, p. 978; Slagle, 1990). Because persons with MTBI are highly vulnerable to the potentially adverse effects of medication, medications should be prescribed with caution (NIH, 1999).

Both professionals and nonprofessionals report frustration with women who choose to return to violent relationships despite intervention efforts (Loseke, 1992). Placing this seemingly irrational behavior in the context of MTBI and its effects may help those who work with battered women to manage negative reactions that can interfere with the provision of effective services. For many battered women, it may be a relief to find that some of their symptoms can be explained by neurological rather than, or in addition to, psychological factors and that, with proper diagnosis, they can respond to treatment. Whereas traditional psychosocial interventions may be sufficient for most battered women, for those who manifest symptoms secondary to MTBI, these approaches, although essential, may be insufficient. The goals of empowerment and self-efficacy cannot be accomplished without interventions that address the specific cognitive and psychosocial damage inflicted on battered women as a result of repetitive assaults to the head and face (NIH, 1999). Integration of neurological, psychological, sociological, and environmental factors will broaden our understanding of the problems of battered women and will lead to more informed interventions and improved outcomes.

REFERENCES

American Psychiatric Association. (1994). *Diagnostic and Statistical Manual of Mental Disorders* (4th ed.). Washington, DC: Author.

Bohnen, N., Jolles, J., & Twijnstra, A. (1992). Recovery from visual and acoustic hyperaesthesia after mild head injury in relation to patterns of behavioral dysfunction. *Journal of Neurology, Neurosurgery, and Psychiatry, 55*, 222–224.

Browne, A. (1993). Violence against women by male partners: Prevalence, outcomes, and policy implications. *American Psychologist, 48*, 1077–1087.

Claerhout, S., Elder, J., & Janes, C. (1982). Problem-solving skills of rural battered women. *American Journal of Community Psychology, 10*, 605–612.

Collins, M. W., Grindel, S. H., Lovell, M. R., Dede, D. E., Moser, D. J., & Phalin, B. R. (1999). Relationship between concussion and neuropsychological performance in college football players. *Journal of the American Medical Association, 282*, 964–970.

Dikman, S. S., Temkin, N., & Armsden, G. (1989). Neuropsychological recovery: Relationship to psychosocial functioning and post-concussional complaints. In H. S. Levin, H. M. Eisenberg, & A. L. Benson (Eds.), *Mild head injury* (pp. 229–241). New York: Oxford University Press.

Diller, L. (Ed.). (1992). *Neuropsychological rehabilitation*. New York: Plenum Press.

Eby, K. K., Campbell, J.C., Sullivan, C.M., & Davidson, W.S. (1995). Health effects of experiences of sexual violence for women with abusive partners. *Health Care for Women International, 16*, 563–576.

Ferrant, S. L. (1992). Cognitive processing deficits in battered women: Identification of and relationship to severity of violence. *Dissertation Abstracts International 530*, (UMI No. 9227838) 6B.

Gelles, R. J., & Straus, M. A. (1990). The medical and psychological costs of family violence. In M. A. Straus & R. J. Gelles (Eds.), *Physical violence in American families: Risk factors and adaptations to violence in 8,145 families*. New Brunswick, NJ: Transaction Books.

Gronwall, D. (1989). Cumulative and persisting effects of concussion on attention and cognition. In H. S. Levin, H. M. Eisenberg, & A. L. Benton (Eds.), *Mild head injury* (pp. 153–162). New York: Oxford University Press.

Kay, R., Newman, B., Cavallo, M., Ezrachi, O., & Resnick, M. (1992). Toward a neuropsychological model of functional disability after mild traumatic brain injury. *Neuropsychology, 4*, 371–384.

Kay, T. (1992, October). *Minor TBI: An update on research with clinical issues.* Paper presented at the Pacific Coast Brain Injury Conference, Vancouver, British Columbia, Canada.

Kay, T., Harrington, D., Adams, R., Anderson, T., Berrol, S., & Cicerone, K. (1993). Definition of mild traumatic brain injury. *Journal of Head Trauma Rehabilitation, 8*, 86–87.

Kelly, R. (1975). The posttraumatic syndrome, an iatrogenic disease. *Forensic Science, 6*, 17–24.

Kubzansky, J. D., Kawachi, I., Spiro, A. R., Weiss, S. T., Vokonas, P. S., & Sparrow, D. (1997). Is worrying bad for your heart? A prospective study of worry and coronary heart disease in the Normative Aging Study. *Circulation, 95*, 818–824.

Lawler, K. A., & Terregino, C. A. (1996). Guidelines for evaluation and education of adult patients with mild traumatic brain injuries in an acute care hospital setting. *Journal of Head Trauma Rehabilitation, 11*, 18–28.

Loseke, D. R. (1992). *The battered woman and shelters: The social construction of wife abuse.* Albany: State University of New York Press.

Lovell, M. R., Iverson, G. L., Collins, M. W., McKeag, D. B., & Maroon, J. C. (1999). Does brief loss of consciousness predict neuropsychological decrements following concussion? *Clinical Sports Medicine, 9*, 193–198.

Matser, E. J. T., Kessels, A. G., Lezak, M. D., Jordan, B. D., & Troost, J. (1999, September). Neuropsychological impairment in amateur soccer players. *Journal of the American Medical Association, 282*, 971–973.

National Institutes of Health. (1999, September). Rehabilitation of persons with traumatic brain injury. *Journal of the American Medical Association, 282*, 974–983.

Ochs, H. A., Neuenschwander, M. C., & Dodson, T. B. (1996, June). Are head, neck and facial injuries markers of domestic violence? *Journal of the American Dental Association, 127*, 757–761.

Pelcovitz, D., van der Kolk, B., Roth, S., Mandel, F., Kaplan, S., & Resick, P. (1997). Development of a criteria set and a structured interview for disorders of extreme stress (SIDES). *Journal of Traumatic Stress, 10*, 3–16.

Picard, N., Scarisbrick, R., & Paluck, R. (1999, September). *HELPS* ([Grant No. H128A0002]. Washington, DC: U.S. Department of Education Rehabilitation Services Administration, International Center for the Disabled [TBI-NET]).

Powell, J. W., & Barber-Foss, K. D. (1999). Traumatic brain injury in high school athletes. *Journal of the American Medical Association, 282*, 958–963.

Rosenbaum, A., Hoge, S. K., Adelman, S. A., Warnken, W. J., Fletcher, K. E., & Kane, R. L. (1994). Head injury in partner-abusive men. *Journal of Consulting and Clinical Psychology, 62,* 1187–1198.

Sato, R. A., & Heiby, I. M. (1992). Correlates of depressive symptoms among battered women. *Journal of Family Violence, 7,* 229–245.

Silver, J. M., Hales, R. E., & Yudofsky, S. C. (1994). Neuropsychiatric aspects of traumatic brain injury. In S. C. Yudofsky & R. E. Hales (Eds.), *Synopsis of neuropsychiatry* (pp. 279–306). Washington, DC: American Psychiatric Press.

Silver, J. M., Yudofsky, S. C., & Hales, R. E. (Ed.). (1994). *Neuropsychiatry of traumatic brain injury.* Washington, DC: American Psychiatric Press.

Slagle, D. A. (1990). Psychiatric disorders following closed head injury: An overview of biopsychosocial factors in their etiology and management. *International Journal of Psychiatry in Medicine, 20,* 1–35.

Southern, J. P., Smith, R. M., & Palmer, S. R. (1990). Bird attack on milk bottles: Possible mode of transmission of Campylobacter jejuni to man. *Lancet, 336,* 1425–1427.

Stark, E., & Flitcraft, A. (1996, January). *Testimony to the Attorney General's Task Force on Family Violence.* New York: Department of Justice.

Straus, M. A. (1990). *Manual for the Conflict Tactics Scale (CTS).* Durham: University of New Hampshire.

Straus, M. A., & Gelles, R. J. (1986). Societal change and change in family violence from 1975 to 1985 as revealed in two national surveys. *Journal of Marriage and the Family, 48,* 465–479.

Sutherland, C., Bybee, D., & Sullivan, C. (1998). The long-term effects of battering on women's health. *Women's Health: Research on Gender, Behavior, and Policy, 4,* 41–70.

Teasdale, G., & Jennet, B. (1974). Assessment of coma and impaired consciousness: A practical scale. *Lancet, 2,* 81–83.

Walker, L. E. (1977–1978). Battered women and learned helplessness. *Victimology: An International Journal, 2,* 525–534.

Walker, L. E. (1991, Spring). Post-traumatic stress disorder in women: Diagnosis and treatment of battered woman syndrome. *Psychotherapy, 28,* 21–29.

Walker, L. E. (1994). The battered woman syndrome is a psychological consequence of abuse. In R. J. Gelles & D. R. Loseke (Eds.), *Current controversies on family violence* (pp. 133–153). Newbury Park, CA: Sage.

Wilt, S. A., Illman, S. M., & Field, M. B. (1997). *Female homicide victims in New York City: 1990–1994.* New York: Department of Health, Injury Prevention Program.

EPILOGUE:
WHERE DO WE GO FROM HERE?

KATHLEEN A. KENDALL-TACKETT

I recently conducted an in-service training for the family practice residents at our local hospital. The topic was the health care needs of adult survivors of childhood abuse. In talking with them, I was startled to realize that these young physicians, right out of medical school, were not familiar with the myriad studies documenting the behavioral and psychological aspects of health; knowledge that is critical when working with this vulnerable population.

Family violence has the potential to be the bridge that joins the worlds of physical and mental health, because it leaves in its wake symptoms that are both physical and psychological. It is impossible to successfully treat these patients without an approach that integrates both.

Yet, there is much that we still do not know. Let's consider the issue of race. Chapter 3 described the experiences of women of color in abusive relationships, and chapter 8 raised the question of race in an aging population. However, race and ethnicity need even further integration into what is known about family violence and health. For example, we know that racism can have a negative impact on health (Clark, Anderson, Clark, & Williams, 1999), so the next question we need to ask is how racism and social stratification intersect with trauma. Do they compound the effects? What unique strengths and resiliency factors do various cultures provide?

We can raise similar questions about other populations, including people with disabilities, sexual minorities, and low-income people. To what extent are these populations more (or less) vulnerable, and how does the experience of family violence influence their health and well-being?

Finally, we need to better delineate the mechanisms by which family violence leads to illness. Beyond injury, why does family violence make people sick? To answer this question, we can draw from the literature on chronic stress. We can integrate findings on the impact of social relationships on wellness. We can talk about depression and posttraumatic stress disorder not only as outcome variables but also as mechanisms that lead to poor health. We can also talk about the role of beliefs—how these are affected by abuse, how they may make people stay in abusive situations, and how beliefs can either compromise health or lead to healing (Kendall-Tackett, 2003).

These are goals for the future. In the meantime, there are some specific steps you can take with the patients you are seeing now.

WHAT YOU CAN DO NOW

Take a Complete History That Includes All Types of Abuse

There is an axiom in survey research that says "ask what you want to know." This is a useful principle in clinical practice as well. Keep in mind that patients may initially tell you "no," even when there is ongoing or past abuse. This is not surprising, given that many abuse survivors are mistrustful (Kendall-Tackett, 2003). However, you can leave the door open for them to discuss this with you at a future point.

Form Alliances With Other Professionals to Provide Comprehensive Treatment

If you have not already done so, it's time to get out of the professional ghetto and start working collaboratively with other health care providers. That means forming alliances between medical and mental health professionals. It also means finding out about physical health problems in your mental health clients and asking about life circumstances in patients you see for medical care. Only by doing this can these patients be adequately served.

Be Careful in How You Present the Psychological Component of Treatment to Patients

Many abuse survivors are in poor health and have been bounced around the health care system. They have often been told that their symptoms are not "real." Some of these patients may be sent to you. Make sure that patients know that you think they are presenting a true illness, then explain how you think the psychological component will help.

Be Explicit About How You Intend to Use the Information You Collect

Patients are often very concerned that others do not find out about past or current abuse. Unfortunately, medical records are not always confidential. If you want patients to open up to you, you must treat their information with care. Never record any information about family violence on insurance forms, as these can go to the patient's employer.

Even If Abuse Is Involved, Don't Attribute All Symptoms to It

Once you recognize the health impact of family violence, you must be careful not to fall into the trap of assuming that all symptoms are related to it. An abuse survivor I know was in a car accident. Her physician attributed all her current symptoms to her abuse experience. However, the symptoms did not remit, even after hypnosis. It turned out that she had a concussion. Chapter 12 also vividly illustrates the danger allegorizing physical symptoms. Clinicians must be balanced in their approach and acknowledge that abuse can cause health problems, but must not swing the other way and attribute everything to it.

Practice Professional Self-Care

Finally, as you work with this population of patients, it's very important that you practice professional self-care. Asking about family violence makes you privy to some very disturbing secrets. There are two phenomena you should watch for: (a) vicarious traumatization and (b) countertransference. Vicarious traumatization occurs when one becomes traumatized by learning about the abuse experiences of others. It can, not surprisingly, lead to severe personal distress (Friedman, 2001). Vicarious traumatization appears to be relatively common among individuals who work with abuse survivors. For example, in a national study of 1,000 female psychotherapists, those with the highest levels of exposure to sexual abuse material had the highest levels of trauma symptoms (Brady, Guy, Poelstra, & Brokaw, 1999).

Countertransference happens when a patient's story triggers memories of abuse in the clinician. Countertransference is more likely to occur when patients reveal histories that are similar to the clinician's own story (Friedman, 2001). As Hamberger and Patel described in chapter 4, it can also be a barrier to screening for abuse among health care providers.

Abuse histories are fairly common in both mental and medical health care providers. For example, in a survey of 645 professionals who conduct sexual abuse evaluations, 17% reported a history of sexual abuse, and 7% reported a history of physical abuse (Nuttall & Jackson, 1994). In another study of 501 clinicians, Little and Hamby (1996) found that 32% reported a history of child sexual abuse. Therapists who had been sexually abused reported more difficulties with countertransference and boundary issues.

How to Practice Self-Care

As you work with this population, it's important to take some steps to prevent vicarious traumatization and countertransference.

Don't go it alone. Get some help. Realize that most of these patients will benefit from a team of health care professionals. Start forming collaborative relationships with others. This can include having regular supervision if you are in training. Also, if a patient's story is stirring up some memories in you, don't be afraid to seek counseling yourself.

Limit your involvement. Train yourself not to carry your patients' concerns once you leave the office. Keep firm boundaries between your work and home life. This way, you can continue to be connected and caring in the office while minimizing the emotional toll of this type of caring. Another strategy is to limit the number of trauma cases that you see. Try to balance out your caseload with less severely affected patients.

Take care of your body and soul. This final strategy is especially important. It means getting enough sleep, eating nutritious foods, exercising, connecting with others, and maintaining a spiritual life. If you are going to continue in this work, you must take time to rest and replenish.

CONCLUSION

I hope the chapters in this volume have encouraged you to work with this population of patients. These patients are frequent users of health care services but ones who receive inadequate or ineffective care. They need what you have to offer. The chapter authors and I wish you the very best in this important work.

REFERENCES

Brady, J. L., Guy, J. D., Poelstra, P. L., & Brokaw, B. F. (1999). Vicarious traumatization, spirituality, and the treatment of sexual abuse survivors: A national survey of women psychotherapists. *Professional Psychology: Research and Practice, 30,* 386–393.

Clark, R., Anderson, N. B., Clark, V. R., & Williams, D. R. (1999). Racism as a stressor for African Americans: A biopsychosocial model. *American Psychologist, 54,* 805–816.

Friedman, M. J. (2001). *Posttraumatic stress disorder: The latest assessment and treatment strategies.* Kansas City, MO: Compact Clinicals.

Kendall-Tackett, K. A. (2003). *Treating the lifetime health effects of childhood abuse: A guide for mental health, medical and social service professionals.* New York: Civic Research Institute.

Little, L., & Hamby, S. (1996). Impact of a clinician's sexual abuse history, gender, and theoretical orientation on treatment issues related to childhood sexual abuse. *Professional Psychology: Research & Practice, 27,* 617–625.

Nuttall, R., & Jackson, H. (1994). Personal history of childhood abuse among clinicians. *Child Abuse & Neglect, 18,* 455–472.

AUTHOR INDEX

Numbers in italics refer to listings in the reference sections.

SUBJECT INDEX

risk of abuse for, 99–100
societal contributions to risk for, 101
treatment issues for, 103–105
and victimization, 98
Child sexual abuse, 38
estimates of, 82
in health care providers' histories, 250
Chinese-American women, 55
Chronic bronchitis, 4
Chronic disease, 4, 82
Chronic exposure to family violence, 104
Chronic hyperarousal, 39, 144
Chronic illness, 39
Chronic low back pain, 156
Chronic pain, 4, 11, 155–173
assessment of, 167–168
biomedical/biopsychosocial models of, 157–158
and chronic psychological stress, 160
cognitive–behavioral therapy for trauma and, 164–172
and collaborative health care, 171–172
education about, 169
generalization and maintenance of, 170–171
guide to integrating PTSD treatment and, 163–164
individualized treatment planning for, 168
integrative model of, 160–163
and physical injury, 159–160
and PSTD assessment, 165–166
and skill acquisition/rehearsal, 169–170
syndromes of, 156
and trauma, 159–163
Chronic pelvic pain, 11, 159
Chronic psychological stress, 160
Circular burns, 115
Clark, R., 144
Clark, V. R., 144
Cocaine, 189
Cognition
abilities of, 142
achievements with, 13
chronic pain and demands on, 160
distortions of, 235
loss of abilities for, 133
problems with, 137

Cognitive Appraisal of Risky Events, 181
Cognitive–behavioral therapy (CBT), 164–172, 189
Cognitive deficits, 234
Cognitively impaired individuals, 19–20
Cognitive processing therapy, 186
Cohen, T., 138
Collaboration, 103, 105, 250
in childbearing, 212
in chronic pain management, 156, 163, 171–172
Collins, M. W., 235
Comas-Diaz, L., 56
Comfort, client's, 186
Communication
with deaf children, 96–97
with disabled children, 102
doctor–patient, 73
of fears, 38
and prenatal medical procedures, 201
sexual, 191
unwillingness for, 40
of victim-friendly environment, 76
Communication disorders, 97, 98, 104
Community agencies, 186
Community centers, 17
Community response teams, 15
Community services, 116
Compassion, 74
Compassion fatigue, 98
Competency evaluations, 18, 110
Complex posttraumatic stress disorder, 225–226
Complex trauma, 225–226
Compliance, 186
Concentration, 137, 234–236, 239
"Concurrent Treatment of PTSD and Cocaine Dependence" (Back, Dansky, Carroll, Foa, & Brady), 188, 189
Concussions, 139, 235
Conditioned fears, 160
Conditioning, 162
Condom use, 11–12
Conduct disorders, 98
Confidentiality, 13, 19, 65, 113, 172, 248
Conflict Tactics Scale, 40
Confusion, 113, 235, 239
Congestive heart failure, 134
Connecting with others, 250

Evasiveness, 40
Examinations
    pelvic, 201
    physical, 168, 185, 186
    vaginal, 205
Excessive fetal growth, 199
Exclusion, 97
Exercise, 250
Expectations, 72–73
Expected unchangeability of life stress
    (EU), 140
Experience
    awareness of physical, 224
    birth, 208
    peer, 141
    pregnancy, 198–199
Exploratory surgery, 36–37
Exposure
    during breast-feeding, 210
    during labor and delivery, 205
Expressive-writing programs, 89, 90
Eye contact, 223
Eyeglasses, 115, 133
Eyes. *See* Vision

Fabiano, P. M., 191
Facial injuries, 182, 235
Facial lacerations, 35
Failure to protect children, 20
Failure to thrive, 22, 104
Faith, sense of, 220
Falls, 112, 134
False teeth, 115
Family Health History, 85
Family(-ies)
    of children with disabilities, 100–
        101
    disruption of roles of, 57
    elder abuse by, 115–118
    milestones of, 131
    need to preserve the, 47
    postpartum relationships of, 207–208
    as term, 9
Family practitioners, 212
Family violence, 3–5
    assessment of, 13–16
    and chronic pain, 164–172
    coordinated community response to,
        16–17
    documentation issues with, 17–19

    dynamics of, 20–23
    education about, 66–67
    and health, 3–4
    health consequences of, 9, 11–13
    legal issues for specific, 19–20
    mental health providers' role in, 4
    overlapping types of, 15
    summary of, 10–11
    types of, 8
Fatalism, cultural, 56
Fatigue, 36, 37, 156, 235
Fear
    of abandonment, 104
    of care-providers, 118
    communication of, 38
    of disclosure, 102
    of discrimination, 48
    and dissociation, 220
    in ethnic minority women, 47
    of falling, 134
    of legal consequences, 48
    of loss of children, 48, 50, 71
    of loss of control, 34, 68–69, 71, 74
    normal responses of, 160–161
    of offending patients, 67, 74
    in older adults, 111
    and relational trauma psychotherapy,
        221, 222
    of retaliation, 104
    of retribution, 70–71
    of sex, 12
    of surgery, 34
    therapists' feelings of, 216
Fearfulness, 34
Feedback
    on behavioral rehearsals, 169
    on patient outcomes, 73, 75
Feeling "out of it," 239
Felitti, V. J., 227
Fetal growth, excessive, 199
Fetal movement, 199
Fetus, effects on the, 12
Fibromyalgia, 156
Filing for separation or divorce, 53
Financial exploitation, 111, 119
Financial issues, 53, 71, 118
Financial management, 113
Financial stress, 236
Flashbacks, 38, 204, 205, 209, 216, 225
"Forced" living situations, 120, 121
Forced penetration, 205

Forced sexual intercourse, 35, 38
Forgetting appointments, 239
Fractures, 4, 35, 112, 182, 227
Frailty, 113
Frawley, M. G., 223
Freud, Sigmund, 219
Friedman, M. J., 227
Functional aids, 115
Futility, sense of, 71–72
Future orientation, 144

Gagen, D., 70
Gastroenterology services, 36
Gastrointestinal pain, 159
Gastrointestinal symptoms, 138
Gate control theory, 157–158, 169
Gay people, 143
Gender differences
    in abuse of children with disabilities,
        100
    in abuse reports, 86–87
    in elder abuse, 110, 119
    in power, 21
    in quality of life reporting, 87–88
Generalization phase (of chronic pain),
    170–171
Genitals
    injuries to, 182
    lacerations around the, 112
Gerbert, B., 41, 74
Gidycz, C. A., 191
Ginzburg, K., 136, 137
Glaser, R., 39
Glasgow Coma Scale, 237
Glaucoma, 133
Goodwin, J. M., 222, 227
Goodwin, M. M., 73
Gottesman, I. I., 143
Grady, D., 36
Greenwald, S., 139
Griffin, E., 75
Group cognitive–behavioral treatment,
    189
Grumbach, K., 69
Guardians, 19
Guided imagery, 184
Guilt
    and breastfeeding, 210
    in children with disabilities, 105

and elder abuse, 111, 116
and risky behavior, 181, 185
Gulf War, 137
Guse, C., 69
Gynecological examinations, 186

HAC (Health Appraisal Clinic), 84
Haley, W., 142
Hamberger, L. K., 66, 67, 69, 74, 75
Hamby, S., 250
Hamel-Bissell, B. P., 141
Hanscom, K. L., 143
Hansen, M., 70
Hanson-Breitenbecher, K. A., 191
Harel, Z., 137
Harvard Heart Letter, 136
Harway, M., 70
Harwell, T. S., 75
Headaches, 11, 156, 159, 235, 239
Head injuries, 139, 182, 235
Head trauma, 233–244. *See also* Mild
    traumatic brain injury
    and battered women survey, 236–
        242
    effects of, 236
    implications of, 242–244
    screening for, 236, 237, 242–243
    symptoms of, 234–235
Healing, 39
Health Appraisal Clinic (HAC), 84
Health care providers, 63–77
    abuse awareness in, 41
    abuse history of, 250
    abuse screening by, 65–66
    attitudes/accountability of, 69
    barriers of, 66–69
    and CCR model, 16
    and children with disabilities, 101
    choosing perinatal, 199–200
    control of patient relationship by,
        68–69, 74
    discomfort of, 69–70
    for elderly patients, 142–143
    and expectation barriers, 72–73
    family violence summary for, 10–11
    and fear of offending patients, 67, 74
    lack of knowledge of, 66–67
    and patient barriers, 70–72
    perceived irrelevance of IPV to, 68
    and perceived time pressures, 67–68

Intimate partner violence (IPV), 35–37, 39–41
   health care provider barriers to discussion of, 66–69
   patient barriers to discussion of, 70–72
   system-level barriers to screening of, 70–72
Intrapsychic defense, 224
Inui, T., 66
In vivo exposure interventions, 170
Involvement, limiting, 250
IPV. *See* Intimate partner violence
Irrelevance of domestic violence, perceived, 68
Irritability, 137, 235
Irritable bowel syndrome, 11
Ischemic heart disease, 4, 183
Isolation
   of children with disabilities, 101, 102, 104
   of ethnic minority women, 47, 56, 57
   and giving up driving, 133
   and head trauma, 235
   of older people, 111, 112, 121
   reducing, 243
Israel, 137
Iverson, G. L., 235

James, J., 142
Jasinski, J. L., 56
JCAHO (Joint Commission for the Accreditation of Healthcare Organizations), 49
Joint Commission for the Accreditation of Healthcare Organizations (JCAHO), 49
Joint interviews, 124
Joking, 69
Judgment, poor, 235, 236
Juvenile offenders, 16
Juvenile rheumatoid arthritis, 97

Kaiser Permanente, 84, 89
Kaufman Kantor, G., 56
Kendall-Tackett, K. A., 39
Kidnapping, 20, 100
Kidney, 35

Kilpatrick, D. G., 182
Kinesthesis, 134
Knowledge, lack of, 66–67
Knutson, J., 96
Knutson, J. F., 97, 100
Koverola, C., 56
Kraaij, V. W. de, 137
Kramer, R., 139
Krauss, M. W., 141
Kurz, D., 75

Labor and delivery (childbearing), 68, 203–206
Lacerations, 112
Lactation consultants, 209–210, 212
Laferriere, R. H., 141
LaFromboise, T. D., 56
La Leche League, 210
Lane, P. L., 38
Language
   and auditory changes, 133
   as barrier, 48
   of client, 52, 53
   deficits in, 236
   delays in, 104
   disabilities of, 97, 100
Larkin, G. L., 69
Late-onset spousal abuse, 117
Latina women, 47
Launching of children, 131
Law enforcement
   and CCR model, 11, 17
   intervention by, 13, 15, 16
   in support network, 186
Lawrence, J. M., 73
Lawrence, S., 69
Learned helplessness, 111
Learning disabilities, 97, 101
Left-hemisphere deficits, 104
Legal issues
   for cognitively impaired individuals, 19–20
   ethnic minority residency as, 50
   medical records as documentation in, 17–18
   with parental discipline, 21
   resources for, 53
   risk behaviors leading to, 183
Legs, 182
Lesbians, 143

Prison time by a family member, 86
Privacy, 13–14, 18–19
Probabilism, 143
Problem-solving abilities, 170, 235, 236
Progressive diseases, 156
Progressive muscle relaxation, 184
Prolonged-exposure techniques, 168, 170, 186
Protection
    failure to provide, 20
    from head injury, 243
    from the perpetrator, 13–14
    of potential victims, 16
"Protective" partners, 40
Protective services, 15
    child, 13, 17, 71
    elder, 114, 124, 125
Protocols, screening, 73, 75, 172
Pseudoseizures, 104
Psychiatric services, 37, 52
Psychobiological effects, 226
Psychodynamic therapy, 219
Psychoeducation, 184–185, 221
Psychological abuse, 111
Psychological needs, 221
Psychological stress, 160
Psychological symptoms of abuse, 37–38, 47
Psychological tasks (of pregnancy), 201–203
Psychologists, 163, 164
Psychosis, postpartum, 208
Psychosomatic symptoms, 22
Psychotropic medication, 143, 203
PTSD. See Posttraumatic stress disorder
Puerto Ricans, 56

Quality of life, 87–88
Quebec Health Survey, 143

Racism, 46, 48, 54–55, 144
Rage, 216
Rape
    labor and delivery similar to, 205
    and physical abuse, 8
    pregnancy resulting from, 11
    and STDs, 182
Rape crisis centers, 186
Raphael, B., 73

Reaffimation, 41
Reasoning biases, 160
Recidivism, 183
Recovery from surgery, 37, 38
Re-enactment, 222, 223
Referral networks, 73, 90
Referrals, 186
Regulation of affect, 23, 104, 160, 184, 223, 225
Rehabilitation treatment, 243
Rehearsals
    and chronic pain, 169–170
    communication, 201
Relapses, 170–171, 183
Relational trauma therapy, 217–225
Relationship(s)
    abuse in multiple, 15–16
    attachment wounds in, 221
    breastfeeding, 210
    difficulties with, 137, 225
    with mother, 203, 207
    nature of intimate, 72
    with perinatal health care provider, 200
    in postpartum period, 207–208
    with preceding generation, 131
    and pregnancy, 202–203
    previous success in, 141
Relaxation techniques, 143, 170, 184, 201
Religion, 48, 220
Reliving of violent events, 216
Reporting
    of abuse of children with disabilities, 102
    of elder abuse, 113–114, 124
    mandatory obligations for, 13, 15
Research, physical health, 225–228
Residential homes, 97
Resources
    access to, 183
    childbearing, 212, 213
    information about, 243
    lack of social/economic, 130
    legal, 53
    women's centers as, 65
Respect, 52, 74, 221
Respite care, 98
Response of relatives, 16
Responsibility
    accepting, xii, 74, 90, 103

Self-medication, 144, 199
Self-monitoring, 167
Self-neglecting older people, 109–112, 118
Self-protective strategies, 105
Self-regulation, 104
Self-soothing behaviors, 216
Self-worth, 115, 221, 223
Seltzer, M. M., 141
Sensitization, 160, 161
Sensory changes, 134
Sensory impairment, 227
Sensory memories, 216
Separation, legal, 53, 86
September 11, 2001 terrorist attacks, 136
Sexism, 54
Sexual abuse
    child, 38, 82, 250
    of children with disabilities, 100
    and dissociation, 216
    of elderly people, 122–123
    gender differences in, 86
    in health care providers' histories, 250
    health consequences of, 11–12
    injuries from, 182
    as negative life event, 137
    of older people, 111
Sexual assault prevention programs, 191
Sexual behavior, 235
Sexual communication, 191
Sexual dysfunction, 236
Sexual intercourse, 35, 36, 38
Sexual interest, decreased, 12
Sexuality, 199, 202, 221
Sexually transmitted diseases (STDs)
    in adult survivors of childhood abuse, 83
    and dissociation, 227
    and elder abuse, 112
    and rape, 11
    and risky behavior, 180
    from sexual assault, 182
    testing for, 186
    in women, 36
Sexual partners, number of, 227
Sexual talk, 100
SF-36. *See* Medical Outcome Study Short-Form 36-Item Health Survey

Shaken baby syndrome, 98
Shaking, severe, 237, 240
Shame
    and breastfeeding, 210
    and culture, 55, 56
    and dissociation, 217, 220, 221, 226
    and elder abuse, 111
    in postpartum period, 208
    and pregnancy, 202
    and risky behavior, 181, 185
Shelters. *See* Domestic violence shelters
Short, L. M., 66
Sibling assault, 9
Siegel, J. A., 138
Silver, J. M., 139
Simultaneous treatments, 188
Single-parent status, 100
Situational reappraisals, 141
Skeletal fractures, 4, 183
Skills
    for chronic pain management, 169–170
    communication, 102
    level of, 48
Skin conditions, 112
Skull trauma, 35
Sleep/sleep disorders, 22, 130, 133, 137, 156, 235, 250
Smell acuity, 134
Smith, D. W., 184
Smoking, 82, 83, 199, 227
Social behavior, 235
Social networks, 141
Social norms, exposure to different, 48
Social service systems, 101
Social support, 47
Societal attitudes, 101
Soft-tissue pain, 36
Sohi, B. K., 56
Solomon, Z., 136, 137
Somatization, 37, 219, 225, 226
Sore nipples, 209
Space, physical, 73
Speech disabilities, 97, 100, 104
Spinal cord, 104, 157–158
Spine deformities, 227
Spirituality, 221
Spiritual life, 220, 250
Spitz, A. M., 73
Spitznagel, E. L., 138
Spleen, 35

Splintered Reflections (Goodwin & Attias), 227
Spontaneity, 235
Spontaneous abortion, 199
Spouses (as elder abusers), 115–117
Statutes of limitations, delayed-discovery, 144
STDs. *See* Sexually transmitted diseases
"Stirrups" position, 34
Stone Center, 221
Straus, M. A., 40
Stress
    and chronic pain, 158, 159, 165
    chronic psychological, 160
    of ethnic minority women, 57
    on families of children with disabilities, 98
    health-related, 135
    and wound healing, 39
Stress hormones, 38, 39, 144, 160
Stress–illness linkage, 37–39
Stress-induced analgesia, 226–227
Stress inoculation therapy, 168, 186
Stroke, 4, 135
Substance abuse
    and brain injury, 236
    and chronic pain, 156
    and dissociation, 227
    and elder abuse, 112, 115, 117, 118
    evaluation for, 186
    gender differences in, 86
    and PTSD, 187–189
    and risky behavior, 180, 181
"Substance Dependence PTSD Therapy" (Triffleman, Carroll, & Kellogg), 188
Successful aging, 141
Sugg, N. K., 66
Suicide/suicidal thoughts, 37, 139, 236
Suitor, J. J., 141
Sullivan, P., 96
Sullivan, P. M., 97, 100
Supervision, 250
Support
    age mate, 137
    birth, 204
    breastfeeding, 209–211
    for chronic pain management, 170, 171
    from colleagues, 217
    for elderly trauma survivors, 141–142

    emotional, 243
    postpartum, 207, 209
    and risky behaviors, 184
    social, 47
    systemic, 73
Support groups
    for ethnic minority women, 52
    infertility, 211
Supportive environment
    for ethnic minority women, 52
    for surgery, 41
Surgeon General's report, 46, 47
Surgery(-ies), 33–41
    and adult survivors of childhood abuse, 36
    and anxiety, 38
    and awareness of abuse, 41
    exploratory, 36–37
    individual abuse history and number of, 35
    and interventions, 38–39
    and psychological symptoms of abuse, 37–38
    recovery from, 37
    screening for family violence before, 34–35
    and screening for violence, 40–41
    supportive environment for, 41
    and women's victimization history, 36–37
Symptoms of abuse
    in adult survivors, 36
    medical record of, 18
    in Mexican-American women, 47
    physical, 18, 35–36, 40, 47
    psychological, 37–38, 47
    unexplained, 40
Synapses, 133
System-level barriers, 73–76

Taste, 134
TBI. *See* Traumatic brain injury
T-cells, 39
Teachers, 99, 101
Teams, community response, 15, 16–17
Tears, 223
Teen pregnancy, 83
Temperature, body, 133
Tension reduction behavior, 181
Terror attacks, 38, 216

Virtual sex, 100
Vision, 47, 97, 132, 133
Visual imagery, 216
Vulnerability
    in childbearing, 197
    to chronic pain, 162
    of elderly victims, 113

Waalen, J., 73
Waking the Tiger (Levine), 227
Walker, E. A., 83
Walker, L. E., 234
Wechsler Adult Intelligence Scale–
    Revised, 142
Weiner, H., 227
Weissman, M., 139
Welfare assistance, 18
Welfel, E. R., 114
White, J. L., 54
Widows, 141
Wiens, A. G., 38
Williams, D. R., 144
Williams, L. M., 138
Winterbauer, N., 70
Wisconsin Department of Health and
    Social Services, 111

Witnessing, 22–23
Women
    of childbearing age, 12
    and head trauma. *See* Head trauma
    number of injuries to, 3
    number of partner assaults on, 234
    preoperative anxiety in, 38
    risky behaviors of, 183, 185
    support networks for, 141
Women's resource centers, 65
Wong, J., 138
Work absences, 236
Workforce milestones, 132
Workloads, high, 73
World Health Organization, 3, 111
Worldview, 221–222
World War II veterans, 139
Wound healing, 39
Writing programs, 89, 90
Wukasch, R. N., 37

Yeast infections, 47

Zaccaro, D., 69
Zaslav, M. R., 188
Zero-tolerance programs, 101

ABOUT THE EDITOR

Kathleen A. Kendall-Tackett, PhD, is a health psychologist, an international board certified lactation consultant, and a research associate professor of psychology at the Family Research Lab at the University of New Hampshire. Her work focuses on two main areas of study: family violence and perinatal health. Her current research interests include the long-term health effects of childhood abuse, the impact of maternal depression, and the psychological aspects of breastfeeding. Dr. Kendall-Tackett is a fellow of Division 38 (Health Psychology) of the American Psychological Association, and is the author or editor of six books, including *Treating the Long-Term Health Effects of Childhood Abuse* (2003). She is on the editorial boards of *Child Abuse & Neglect* and the *Journal of Child Sexual Abuse,* and has served as program cochair for the International Family Violence Research Conferences since 2000.

Dr. Kendall-Tackett has won several awards including the Outstanding Research Study Award from the American Professional Society on the Abuse of Children; most recently, she was named 2003 Distinguished Alumna, College of Behavioral and Social Sciences, California State University, Chico.

She lives in New Hampshire with her husband Doug, her sons Ken and Chris, and quite a few pets.